D0868512

THE
Mindful
BODY

THE
Mindful
BODY

BUILD EMOTIONAL STRENGTH
AND MANAGE STRESS WITH
BODY MINDFULNESS

NOA BELLING

INTERNATIONAL BEST-SELLING AUTHOR AND PSYCHOLOGIST

ROCKPOOL
PUBLISHING

Recent scientific research has supported what contemplative practices have known for hundreds and even thousands of years that opening awareness to the signals of the body is a window to wisdom. This wisdom, this source of deep knowing from our internal world, also connects us with empathy for the internal world of others.

DR DANIEL J. SIEGEL

Professor of psychiatry at UCLA School of Medicine,
Executive Director of the Mindsight Institute

A Rockpool book
PO Box 252
Summer Hill
NSW 2130
Australia
www.rockpoolpublishing.com.au
http://www.facebook.com/RockpoolPublishing

Belling, Noa, author.
The mindful body / Noa Belling.
978-1-925682-18-2 (paperback)
Mind and body.
Mindfulness (Psychology).

First published in 2018
Copyright Text © Noa Belling 2018
Copyright Design © Rockpool Publishing 2018

Cover and internal design by Seymour design
Illustrations by Marcella Cheng
Typesetting by Graeme Jones
Printed and bound in China

10 9 8 7 6 5 4 3 2 1

All rights reserved. No part of this publication may be reproduced, stored in
a retrieval system, or transmitted in any form or by any means, electronic,
mechanical, photocopying, recording or otherwise, without the prior written
permission of the publisher.

The author of this book does not dispense medical advice or prescribe the use of
any technique as a form of treatment for physical or mental problems without the
advice of a physician, either directly or indirectly. In the event you use any of the
information in this book, neither the author nor the publisher can assume any
responsibility for your actions. The intent of the author is only to offer information
of a general nature to help in your quest for personal growth.

In this book there are descriptions of personal experiences to illustrate different
aspects of the material being presented. The particulars of individuals have been
changed in order to protect the confidentiality of clients, workshop participants and
students. Any names used are purely fictional.

Contents

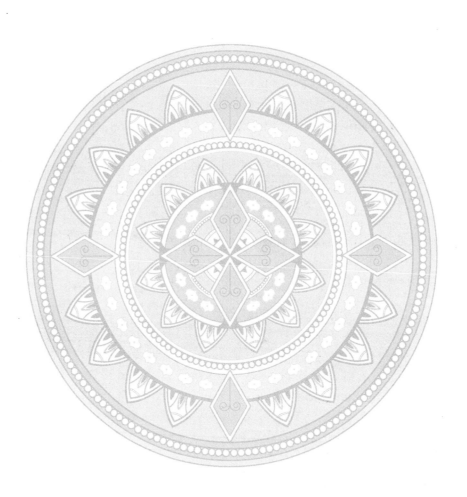

Foreword

Everybody has a body. Everybody *is* a body. A dictionary definition of body is 'the main or central part of anything'. In her method of positioning our bodies as a central part of our healing and our ongoing wellbeing, Noa Belling has joined the ranks of an increasing majority of doctors, therapists, counselors, and educators who include *and* integrate our physical selves into the theory and practice of increasing human potential.

Back in the 1970s, when I was getting started in this field as a dance therapist and bodyworker, the idea that our physical health was closely related to our emotional or cognitive health was a fringe belief. Western medicine practised in an almost completely separate location to psychotherapy, which in turn practised in territories largely distant from physical education. The idea that there was a bi-directional influence between how you moved and your emotional, cognitive, and relational wellbeing, was largely relegated to New Age crackpots.

Over the years I have watched and marveled as our location at the fringe has been migrating towards the centre, to the point where, now, two decades into the 21ˢᵗ century, the assumption of body/mind integration has landed in the mainstream. Physicians are getting some of their most powerful results from the practice of behavioural medicine, a field that urges people to exercise to address mild-to-moderate depression, to notice that what they eat affects not only their blood sugar but their mood, and to ward off cognitive decline by dancing and hanging out with friends.

In the fields of psychotherapy and counseling, similar shifts have occurred. Psychotherapists and counselors began to identify the limitations of Freud's 'Talking Cure'. They have noted that discussing one's past, to gain insight in the hope of producing therapeutic change, yielded poor outcomes or only modest results. This was often after patients had spent years and many thousands of dollars on therapy. These same psychotherapy and counseling professionals began to notice that their clients' wellbeing improved when the therapy became more experiential, by directly feeling and processing emotions during sessions, for instance, as well as seeing their clients' bodily sensations as another voice trying to be heard. Also, forming a bond with their patients increased the likelihood of their patients feeling secure enough to seek change.

Research, particularly in the field of neuroscience, has yielded dramatic breakthroughs in re-centralising the lived experience of the body in current culture. Many studies have demonstrated that our brains read our bodies in order to organise feeling, thinking, and behaviour; body memory lies at the base of much of our dispositions, attitudes, and feelings; and our body's posture, gestures and movements influence how we appraise stimuli and how we respond to them. Clearly, the time has come to move on from outdated beliefs that the mind and body are separate systems.

Noa Belling's book, *The Mindful Body,* clearly, gracefully, and articulately assists us to heal and thrive. Divided into eleven parts, the book deftly weaves together research and theory from multiple disciplines, with integrative ideas and accessible practices. In reading the book, we learn to see our lives and our relationships as embodied experiences, and have ongoing opportunities to feel that embodiment directly as we read. The themes of the book include decision-making, confidence, relationships and zest for life, and they immediately apply to our daily experiences. The 'Mindful Body' practices help us to respond to the book directly. While scaffolded with research, the flesh and blood of the book speaks to how we can move more purposefully and productively in our world.

An example of this is Noa's recurring emphasis on what emotions are, where they come from, and how we can work with them to lead happier lives. Looking through multiple lenses (such as early childhood development, brain structure and chemistry, trauma theory, and social neuroscience), we can see that emotions begin to organise prenatally, that they begin to operate before we are consciously aware of them, and that they are designed to motivate and guide most of our actions, through the moving body. We now know, through these same disciplines, that emotions are frequently shared with others, that regulating emotions can be a social and personal event, and that emotional resiliency is bound with self efficacy, physical health, and loving kindness.

Working from this integrated perspective requires a nuanced and broad set of strategies. One of the strengths of *The Mindful Body* is its use of practices, which span from ancient wisdom traditions to current activities, and the wide array of exercises from the disparate fields of biofeedback, acupressure, dance therapy, meditation, Yoga, somatic psychology, traumatology, dreamwork, and various forms of visualisation. Of particular note is Noa's emphasis on natural movement, where attending to inner body states is combined with conscious movement responses that emerge and inform us. Movement may be the key here – the movement of our body, our emotions, and our thoughts, in ways that keep us engaged, regulated and relational.

As I write this foreword I feel a unique sense of pride that this field has come to such a point of maturity that *The Mindful Body* can be written and read and followed by so many. Part of this pride stems from the fact that many years ago Noa Belling was my student at Naropa University, in the Somatic Psychology program. It is a great joy to witness her, a living embodiment of mind-body integration, centralising the power of her work in the body of this effective and accessible book.

Christine Caldwell, PhD
Author of *Getting Our Bodies Back,* and *Bodyfulness*

Introduction

*Our bodies hold the potency of all
individual and communal exploration,
supplying the juice, the breath, the
concrete reality, and the resiliency
that allow us to track and savor our
development.*

SUSAN APOSHYAN

Your body is a living expression of your mind. It can also be a grounded, empowering and intelligent resource that can support you in many ways. This book is a practical, personal guide for discovering and exploring the body/mind connection. It delves into how your mind lives in your body and how body awareness can help you, if you wish, to change aspects of your life.

Throughout the book you are invited to explore how your body has a mind of its own. Your body is constantly responding to life all the way from noticeable muscular shifts in posture and facial expression to the more subtle level of the cellular and energetic responses to what is going on inside and around you. This response often occurs before your thinking mind has a chance to catch up. Your body makes independent decisions, too, such as in keeping you alive via your heartbeat, your breathing, and many other body systems. Your body also instinctively triggers a survival response such as 'fight or flight' when you are in danger.

Your body has a memory of its own called implicit memory. When we think of memory, we usually think of explicit memory, which involves consciously recalling the factual details or events of our lives (like what we did on the weekend and with whom). This memory helps us to organise ourselves according to time, place and context. It is supported by language that helps us form narratives about our lives. Explicit memory starts in bits and pieces from about two years old and grows with our grasp of language.

Implicit memory is our non-verbal, feeling-based record of past experience. It is the first memory system in place before we begin to talk and it remains active throughout our lives, beneath our explicit narratives that we add along the way.

Implicit memory has a procedural component and an emotional component.

Procedural

On a procedural level, it kicks in when we experience automatic reactions that do not require focused attention or speech. Riding a bicycle is an example. We react to the feeling of being unbalanced, of needing to move forward and keeping the handlebars straight. We do not focus our thoughts and energy on any one thing in particular. Learning to walk is another procedural memory action. Once it is recorded in memory, most of us would have trouble explaining how we do it. It is just there and generally remains with us for a lifetime.

Emotional

The emotional component of implicit memory records our non-verbal, emotional interactions with people and life. The result is an emotional autobiography that we can sense in our bodies as familiar feeling tones. These feeling tones colour and shape our emotional world and our identity and are also stored below the level of conscious awareness, like riding a bicycle. For example, believing that we are shy, anxious, reserved, moody, outgoing, confident or cheerful, is influenced implicitly by our past experiences. This changes how the world appears to each person or, in words attributed to Anais Nin: 'We don't see things as they are, we see them as *we* are.'

As we mature we begin to identify with our thoughts about life and with the explicit storyline about the history of our lives. However, in truth, it is our implicit, emotional memory that is the real driver of our choices and behaviours.

⇒ CHANGE IS POSSIBLE ⇐

Neuroplasticity refers to the brain's ability to rewire itself and form new neural pathways. Scientific findings in this area show that we are able to change on an implicit and explicit level at any age. In his book *The Brain That Changes Itself*, Norman Doidge refers to change and healing as a process of noticing our feelings, uncovering unconscious memory and putting it into words and into context so that it can be better understood. Then we can find proactive and creative ways to help ourselves. In the process, we can 'plastically' re-transcribe even deeply ingrained implicit memories so that they become conscious explicit memories, sometimes for the first time. It takes time and perseverance to achieve lasting change, but it is within our reach.

This book provides many opportunities to explore how the past and present live in our bodies and affect our experiences of life. There are also many opportunities to make positive changes in our brains and lives through body-mind awareness and practising mindfulness in a body-referenced way.

As a path to mindfulness, body awareness offers a natural route. This is because, at its core, mindfulness is about living with greater presence, which is a natural state for our bodies, which are moving in the here and now. It is only our thoughts that can drift off into the past or the future. For example, many mindfulness practices start with attention to body and breathing as a way to anchor awareness in the moment. So your practice of living more mindfully in and through your body, along with all the other benefits of becoming more body mindful, can also yield results common to the practice of traditional mindfulness. Benefits can include improved physical health, brain function and energy levels, reduced stress, increased emotional resilience, increased positive feelings like optimism, joy, contentment and intimacy, decreased negative feelings like depression, anxiety and isolation, and an improved quality of life.

⇒ MINDFUL BODY MOMENTS AND MINDFUL BODY PROCESSES ⇐

In this book your practical opportunities to create lasting, positive change in your brain and body, are offered in two ways:

Mindful Body Moments

Mindful Body Processes

Together they are designed to yield psychological insight, healing and growth, while promoting healthy brain development and qualities of mindfulness for applying to life.

Mindful Body Moments

Mindful Body Moments are short, impactful exercises for body-mind awareness and integration. These are intended to strengthen the muscles of your mindful embodiment in playful, exploratory ways, while naturally promoting resilience, optimal brain functioning and heart-led living.

The invitation is for you to carry this idea of taking Mindful Body Moments forwards into your life. Any time could be a time for a Mindful Body Moment. It could be a break from working at your computer, a gap between meetings, a moment stuck in traffic, when you are waiting in the shopping line, or waiting to pick up your child from school, or in a free moment at home. You can practise any Mindful Body Moment you choose anywhere and anytime, and discreetly, so that no one else notices. All that is required is for you to remember to include a Mindful Body Moment now and again in your day. You can also dedicate a particular time each day to certain practices, if you wish, for increasing the consistency of your mind-body connectedness. As you become accustomed to doing so, hopefully you will come to appreciate and enjoy these moments so that they do not feel like a chore, and instead become moments you look forward to for their enriching, soothing and enlivening effects.

There are many Mindful Body Moment options offered throughout the book. You are invited to read each and then to take your chosen ones forward into your daily life. Including at least one moment each day for body-mind connection will bring the greatest benefits. Let your own experiments and outcomes be your personal motivation.

You might also wish to experiment with one Mindful Body Moment for a period of time to get to know it better, strengthen its effect and then, because you know it well, use it more readily, on-the-spot, in spare moments. Or you might gravitate to a favourite Mindful Body Moment and focus mainly on that one. Alternatively you might wish to try out different ones at different times, which is helpful for keeping your mind-body exploration and integration feeling fresh, new and interesting.

Mindful Body Processes

Mindful Body Processes are opportunities to gain self-awareness in a more in-depth way than taking a Mindful Body Moment. At times it is helpful to carry out this kind of deeper self-reflection to allow for new awareness to dawn and new resources to be developed. For example, this can apply to working with particularly challenging emotions and memories. And these longer processes tend to generate their own Mindful Body Moments that you can practise thereafter to consolidate the outcome.

Mindful Body Dreaming

In the dreams and imagination chapter, the Mindful Body Moments and Mindful Body Processes are referred to, as Mindful Body Dreaming.

⇛ HOW MUCH TO PRACTISE FOR LASTING CHANGE? ⇚

There is no definitive answer about exactly how much practice creates lasting change. However, there is agreement in the fields of psychology and neuroscience that regularly practising positive, new behaviours is key, even if in short bursts. For example, Dr Rick Hanson has estimated that even 30 seconds of practice a few times a day can effectively rewire the brain and ingrain positive changes in life. The key is to really visualise and embody the new positive state. It is important to hold this state in body and mind for long enough to allow the brain to really register it and respond to it by forming new neural connections. This is why it is recommended to consciously hold awareness of a changed state of body and mind for at least 30 seconds. You will be reminded to do so as you move through the practices in the book, so new neural connections and new, positive life habits can be reinforced and developed over time.

⇒ MINDFUL BODY PROCESS ⇐

A dip inside the mind of your body

To get a sense of how your body and mind live together and how you can influence how you feel, pause for a few moments to try out this experience:

No matter how you are feeling, let your awareness dive deep inside your body. Begin to explore what you find. Become curious about how your body is holding your feelings right now. Perhaps you find some parts of your body are tense or tired, restless or out of balance. You might notice the quality of your breathing. No need to change what you find. For now, treat everything simply as information about your state of body and mind. Take a few moments to look around inside. Perhaps a particular body part draws your attention. Or you might have a general sense of how you feel all over.

Be curious. What is your body expressing? How is it reflecting your feelings and thoughts now? Are you holding your head up high and facing the world? Or perhaps you are tense, lopsided, fidgety or collapsed into yourself, or turning some part of yourself away? What could this reflect about your attitudes to your life at this time?

Now consider how you would like to feel. You might think of a quality like kindness, patience, strength or calmness that you feel would be good for you. Then breathe your chosen quality through you, allowing the feeling of it to become you. Become curious about what could help you on a body level. You might take a few deep breaths. You might try on a new posture, perhaps breathing in, stretching out, or bringing some movement to free up areas that feel tight or that need some enlivening. There is always something you can do on a body level. Notice how this process might shift you – how you breathe, feel, think and face the world.

CHAPTER 1
Greeting Your Body

No other form of communication is more universally understood as touch. The compassionate touch of a hand or a reassuring hug can take away our fears, soothe our anxieties, and fill the emptiness of being lonely.

RANDI FINE

When you first meet someone you might shake hands in greeting. To enter this book's journey of perhaps getting to know your body anew, you are invited to start by also extending a tactile kind of greeting to your body. This is as if to say, 'Hello, here you are and here I am with you'. From there the relationship can begin to develop.

As an initial greeting, you are invited to place your hands on your head. Find the place for each hand that feels best, such as front and back, or top and bottom, where the back of your neck meets your head. Or you can hold both sides of your head. Go with what feels right.

What happens to your thoughts as you hold your head? It may look like the gesture of 'oh my goodness, everything feels so overwhelming', but the sensation may feel more like quick and easy relief from mental busy-ness and a welcome return into your warm body senses, allowing you to breathe again.

In our busy lives full of to-do lists, worries, decisions, criticisms and challenges, our attention can get stuck in our heads day in and day out as we try to hold everything together. Stay holding your head for a few more moments while breathing naturally. Deepen your breathing only if it feels natural. Let go when it feels like enough.

Touch is an effective connector of mind and body and this connection can be experienced in an instant. Your skin feels alive, awakening your body senses. Touch is proven to decrease the physiological effects of stress and anxiety, lowering levels of stress hormones like cortisol, lowering blood pressure, and slowing heart rate. It is also found to strengthen the immune system. Nurturing touch stimulates the release of oxytocin, the 'cuddle' or 'love' hormone, which can relax and clear your mind. Oxytocin can also induce a sense of trust and connection, switch off the fight or flight response, provide welcome soothing when you're feeling emotional, and raise the level of other feel-good hormones like endorphins. Touch can also help you to sleep better by drawing your attention from your busy mind, and into your warm body senses.

⇒ SELF-HOLDING ⇐

How would it feel to hold yourself with the same support and care as you would hold a person you love?

We don't always have others around to be in 'touch' with. Also, touch is quite a 'touchy' subject in the way that it reminds us of our relationship with nurturing, body image, boundaries and sexuality. Luckily, in your own hands, you hold the power to achieve noticeable results. Without necessarily knowing it, we touch ourselves many times a day, anyway. We touch our faces, rub our foreheads, fold our arms, play with our hair, touch our necks, rub and squeeze our hands, play with our fingers, place our hands on our hips, rub our lower backs, cross our legs, rub where it hurts, etc. Often through our instinctive touch we are self-soothing or attempting to ground ourselves, even if we are not conscious that we are doing it. As an experiment, next time you become aware that you are touching yourself, you could try continuing, deliberately, and be more conscious of the experience. This chapter is an invitation to use touch consciously.

To follow are some self-holding options for your exploration. They guide you to give attention to different parts of your body and provide you with constantly available ways to self-support. You could use any of them for stress relief, to provide comfort, or simply to connect with yourself and relax at the end of your day. Try them out to find the ones that you like best.

HOW AND HOW LONG TO HOLD

Steadily hold each position for a few seconds, initially, to get a feel for it. If the position resonates with you, hold for as long as feels nourishing. Breathe naturally as you do so. Some positions might feel amazing. Others not right for today. Hold with a firmness or gentleness that feels just right. As you hold, feel warmth and support from your hands. Feel the pulse of life beneath your skin. Wait for a natural shift, such as an organic deep breath or just a sense that you have held for long enough, to let you know when to move on or let go. Explore the holds that you like best and use your favourite holds regularly.

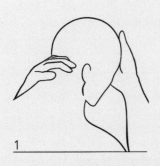

1

THE HOLDS

1. One hand holds the base of your skull (where the back of your head meets the top of your neck). Place your other hand either on the top of your head or over your forehead, whichever feels better for you.

EFFECT: Almost instantly reduces stress, especially where there is mental agitation. Can clear your mind. Shifts your attention to your body senses and allows you to access feelings, which can provide insight into a given situation.

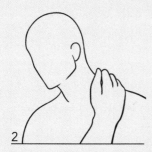

2. One hand gives the opposite trapezius muscle a squeeze. Hold this squeeze for a few breaths. (Your trapezius muscle is between your neck and shoulder and is a common area of tension.) Repeat on the other side. To end, use both hands to rub up and down the back of your neck and over your trapezius area a few times.

EFFECT: Can release your breathing and relieve the sense of carrying the world on your shoulders.

. . . .

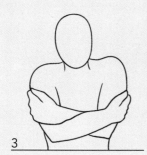

3. Rub your upper arms.

EFFECT: Raises oxytocin or 'cuddle hormone' levels. Helps you sense your personal boundaries.

Hug yourself, either following your natural inclination to wrap your arms around your upper body, or you can slip your hands under your armpits to hold the sides of your upper chest. Relax your elbows at your sides as you hold your hands flat against your ribs and right up under your armpits.

EFFECT: Self love.

. . . .

4. Place one or both of your hands over your heart and hold for a few moments.

EFFECT: Mothers and self-nurtures. Putting a hand on your heart while speaking also displays sincerity and can positively influence how others respond to you.

. . . .

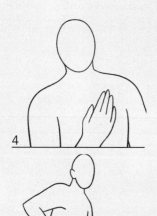

5. Rub your lower back. You could also place one hand on your lower back, behind your hipbone (either side is fine). Place the other hand at the crease of the inner side of your knee on the same side as you are holding your lower back.

EFFECT: Grounds you, energises your legs and encourages a feeling of 'get up and go'.

After holding this position, sweep both hands down your legs, front and back, a few times to enhance the grounding and energising effect.

....

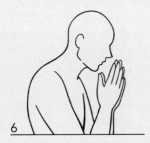

6. Place your hands in a prayer pose, either touching your chest or with a small space between hands and chest, whichever feels better to you.

EFFECT: Centres, reminds of prayer so you can say a little prayer for yourself, too, while holding.

....

End by holding your favourite position and notice how you feel now.

Most of us are so overloaded and busy, whether from work or home life, that a few minutes of self-holding can work wonders. Use the holds that you like whenever you wish. Perhaps you could include some in your bath routine, while lying in bed at night before you go to sleep, or first thing in the morning to set yourself up well for the day. You could add some before or after an exercise routine for some extra body honouring. As you might do for others, you could also simply take hold of your own hand or arm or place a hand on your chest area for support through conflict or challenging moments.

These particular holds are adapted from an acupressure approach called Jin Shin TARA. Jin Shin TARA has its roots in the innately body-mind practice of Chinese Medicine. Guided touch, or holding specific areas of the body, is used as part of a holistic approach to healthcare. Dr Stephanie Mines, founder of the TARA approach, advocates touch as a powerful healing agent for shock and trauma in the body-mind-spirit system. Touch can quickly ground intense feelings. Holding a hand or even just your own finger when you hear shocking news, or when you feel scared, as well as rubbing where it hurts, can provide relief.

THE IDEAL STATE

Finding a balance between the sympathetic and parasympathetic nervous system is key to health and wellbeing.

The sympathetic nervous system

The sympathetic nervous system is characterised by a feeling of energy, alertness and confidence. Out of balance, it could feel like nervousness and agitation, a need to talk rapidly, constriction in the breath, rapid heartbeat, hyperactivity, anxiety, or, in the extreme, panic.

The parasympathetic nervous system

The parasympathetic nervous system is characterised by a feeling of relaxation, connection and introspection. Out of balance it could feel like withdrawal, disconnection, feeling paralysed, shutting down, spaciness, numbness, tiredness or helplessness.

A healthy and creative ideal is characterised by being calmly alert. This combines the best of both the sympathetic and the parasympathetic worlds. Feel-good hormones are released, which uplifts your spirits and promotes health. Touch is a simple and accessible method for supporting yourself to let go of sympathetic or parasympathetic nervous-system extremes and to open to a more balanced, wholesome and grounded state of nervous-system balance.

⇉ ABOUT GREETING OTHERS WITH TOUCH ⇇

In the same way as primates groom each other to strengthen social bonds, human touch also seems to strengthen relationships and foster a sense of closeness and likeability. For example, studies have shown that even fleeting, non-threatening contact with a stranger can have a measurable effect. We are found to be more likely to agree to a request and to respond favourably to a person or a product. This can hold true even when people have no conscious memory of being touched. Touch plays a central and highly influential role throughout our emotional lives whether we are aware of it or not.

According to Tiffany Field, at the Touch Research Institute, the healing power of safe, nurturing touch extends across our life spans. Touch is found to help babies develop a sense of safety and security. Consistent, nurturing touch by parents can help reduce a baby's pain and help them sleep better, reduce their irritability, increase sociability among other infants and improve growth in premature babies. Field has found similar gains later in life, too, such as reduction in chronic pain and improvement in emotional conditions in children and adults when some supportive touch is included regularly in their lives. In the elderly, in addition, Field has found that touch yields emotional and cognitive benefits that can be separated from general social support. In one series of studies, one group of elderly participants received regular, conversation-filled social visits. Another group received social visits that also included massage. The second group recorded more emotional and cognitive benefits than the first.

We also cannot touch without being touched. The physiological benefits of touch, like the rise in oxytocin levels and lowered heart rate, are experienced in both the giver and the receiver. The Touch Research Institute has found that a person giving a massage experiences as great a reduction in stress hormones as the person receiving it. Their studies have also shown that a person giving a hug gets just as much benefit as a person being hugged.

WHEN NOT TO TOUCH

There are people for whom touch does not feel nourishing, however. It can result in resistance and feelings of discomfort. From cultural and religious differences, to personality differences, to family differences and life experience, touch needs to be used sensitively. A rule of thumb if we are using touch with others is to stick to safe zones like the arms and upper back and to be sensitive to the recipient's reaction. Do they warm to your touch or pull away? Respecting this and discontinuing touch if there is resistance, is important. The same applies with those we love. There are times when we are open to each other's physical contact and times we are not. Sensitivity to this involves tuning in to, and respecting, each other's changing needs. Interestingly, according to research, the true indicator of a healthy long-term relationship is not how often each person initiates touch. The true indicator is how often your partner touches you in response to your touch. Laura Guerrero, co-author of *Close Encounters: Communication in Relationships*, says that the more consistently this happens and the stronger the reciprocity, the more likely someone is to report emotional intimacy and satisfaction within the relationship. This touch reciprocity or touch responsiveness can help you to gauge how open a person is to your touch.

⇨ NATURAL SENSE OF BOUNDARY ⇦

Your skin is a natural boundary between you and the outside world. In her book *Natural Intelligence*, body-mind psychotherapist Susan Aposhyan, speaks about using the natural boundary of the skin as a metaphor for healthy psychological boundaries. She applies this in her work with clients who have relationship, nurturing or sexuality issues, and who feel vulnerable in relationships. In her work she encourages touching the skin as a way to wake it and strengthen the experience of a natural boundary.

Take a few moments to wake up the sense of natural boundary that an awareness of your skin can give you. Touch your skin from head to toe (through your clothes where necessary), as if you were soaping yourself in the shower, outlining your skin boundary as you go along. Simply touching your skin can increase your sense of feeling alive. This is part of the reason we can feel so refreshed after a bath or shower.

Your skin is not a boundary that you have to imagine. Rather, it is tangible and real. It offers a readily available psychological boundary that can help you to feel safer in your skin and, by extension, to feel safer in the world.

WHERE THE BOUNDARY BEGINS

The sense of psychological boundary starts developing at the very start of life. In embryos, the skin develops out of the same tissue as the nervous system. Skin remains closely related to the nervous system thereafter, giving it great sensitivity for gathering tactile information about the world. Once we are born our skin also plays a role in the formation of our sense of self. Roz Carroll of the Chiron Body Psychotherapy Centre in London distinguishes between a 'skin ego' (developing on Sigmund Freud's notion of ego) and a 'motoric ego'. Ego refers to a sense of one's 'self' and a sense of one's worth, that is born out of experience. According to Carroll, the skin and motoric egos precede, and lay the foundation for, our adult ego. Our skin ego develops in the first year of life from our experience with touch. Initially the skin ego is felt as physical containment. A newborn baby can experience a bombardment of sensory input that may feel like chaos to his or her newly developing and immature nervous system. The infant is not yet able to sift and sort sensory input. They also cannot distinguish yet between what is from self and what is from their parent or the outside world. Mummy, Daddy or a caregiver comes in with attuned touch and eye contact and it can focus the baby's attention, calming, containing and regulating their nervous system. This supports a baby feeling content and safe in the world and they carry this feeling with them into adulthood. This also translates into the ability to regulate one's own emotions, and models the possibility for relationships being nourishing and supportive. If emotional nurturing is unavailable or inconsistent, the baby can feel emotionally unregulated. Later in life this can present symptoms of being frequently overwhelmed and unable to contain one's emotions, or to feeling emotionally shut down.

The skin ego

Our skin boundary informs where each of us start and where we end. For a baby, touch and being seen and responded to adequately is key to their ability to differentiate what is self and what is not self. This differentiation is also important later in life for forming and maintaining healthy relationships. It forms the foundation for our ability to connect, trust and respond socially as well as providing a foundation for empathy. How comfortable we feel with physical proximity, or closeness and distance to others, also has roots in the first years of life based on our early experiences with proximity. So our skin egos develop out of the intimate contact with our primary caregivers and it is reinforced or shifted through intimate relationships with other people as we grow older and have different kinds of experiences.

The motoric ego

The 'motoric ego' develops after the 'skin ego', once a baby can move about on their own and learn about life through their own initiative and physical exploration. With the motoric ego we learn about influencing the world through our actions to add to the skin ego's experience. Together, the skin and motoric egos form an influential, preverbal foundation for our sense of self as adults. As we grow, our adult egos accumulate more mature perceptions and understandings. Although our original skin and motoric ego imprints remain influential.

⇨ DAILY IDEAS FOR STAYING IN
TOUCH WITH YOUR BODY SELF ⇦

» Use the self-holding options offered at the start of this chapter – once or twice a day, for even a few minutes, to relieve stress and bring some inner peace.

» Pause now and again to notice your body and consider if there is a part that could use some nurturing attention. Perhaps your shoulders feel tight, or your jaw tense, or your back out of alignment. Spend a few moments giving this part of your body a short massage or hold the area in a way that feels supportive. Breathe and stretch into the area. Then move on with your day with your body feeling acknowledged and refreshed.

» Place your right hand on your heart and your left hand on your belly. Find the position that feels best for you. Breathe naturally while holding this position for a few minutes or for as long as feels good. Focus on the warmth from your hands on your body.

» Another area that you can massage is the soft spot at the base of your head, where the back of your neck meets your skull. This is an area that can accumulate tension.

» When you are really feeling overwhelmed or restless, lie down flat on your belly (when you get a chance) with arms and legs where they feel most comfortable. This is an effective way to relax your nervous system towards feeling calmer and clearer. Rest like this for as long as you need to.

» To ease tension in your eyes and mind, rub your hands together, creating warmth, then cup your hands over your closed eyes. Absorb the darkness and warmth deep into your eyes and mind. When you open your eyes again let them be soft in their outlook.

» For an interesting, energising sensation, massage your ears.

» Hug and snuggle with loved ones (including pets) regularly.

» Sharing brief back rubs with a partner or friend is an instant feel-good act. Or you can schedule a massage, for a professional touch.

» Spend time in water to feel held, relaxed and comforted in a womb-like watery way. A bath, spending time in a swimming pool or the sea, or even a shower can do the trick.

» Spend time in the sunshine if it is available to you. Sunrays are therapeutic, positively influencing the chemistry of your brain and the functioning of your body with as little as 30 minutes' exposure a day.

» Give yourself a body brush. Stand up and rub your hands together to warm them. Place your hands on your forehead, then use a continuous brushing stroke as you slide your hands over your head, down the back of your neck, down the sides of your body, round to your lower back and down the backs of your legs (bend your legs if you need to), around the outsides of your legs, and then the insides of your feet, up the insides of your legs, up your abdomen, and then place your hands in a prayer pose. Pause for a moment and then repeat the body brush two more times.

⇉ MINDFUL BODY MOMENT ⇇

Support a part of your body with touch

Pause, at any time during your day, perhaps try it out right now, to bring attention to your body and choose an area that can do with some support through touch and holding. You can follow your instincts or you can choose an option suggested in this chapter. Support your body in your chosen way for at least 30 seconds, or longer if you wish, to allow the effects to really seep into your brain and body before moving back into your day. Repeat now and again throughout the day to produce a positive shift in how you feel and how you approach your work and the people around you.

CHAPTER 2

Brainwaves and the Place for Body Awareness

You and the universe talk in frequencies.
What you think and feel are the frequencies you are sending
and then receiving from the universe.

ROXANA JONES

Every day we transition from sleeping to waking to busy working mode, with different emotions and energy levels passing through us, and then back to resting and sleeping again. These states of consciousness can be represented as brainwave frequencies, mapped using an EEG (an electroencephalograph) and measured in Hertz (cycles per second). They are divided into five bands delineating slow, moderate, and fast brainwaves called Delta, Theta, Alpha, Beta and Gamma.

Our brains cycle through these brainwave states every day and night as a natural part of our human biology. Brainwaves also change according to what we are doing and how we are feeling. When slower brainwaves are dominant we can feel anything from relaxed and calm, to tired, slow and dreamy. When faster brainwaves are dominant we can feel focused and attentive all the way through to feeling wired and hyper-alert. A simplified way of summarising brainwave bands as states of consciousness is, super-thinking and loving (gamma), thinking (beta), light, relaxing and sensing (alpha), emotions and dreaming (theta) and deep relaxation or sleeping (delta).

There is no single brainwave that is 'better' or more 'optimal' than the others. Each serves a purpose. Some help you process and learn new information, others help you calm down after a long, stressful day. Your brain's ability to be flexible and transition through various brainwave frequencies, is key to your energy levels, your ability to focus, how you manage stress, and how well you sleep at night.

If one of the five bands of brainwaves is either over- or under-produced, this state can cause problems. In our fast-paced, modern lives there is a tendency to overuse our beta thinking faculties. With mindfulness, our central command station shifts from thinking to a more energised, present and grounded state of being. It is a gateway to health, creativity and a sense of vitality, while also helping us relax and sleep better at the end of each day.

⇳ BETA BRAINWAVES (12 TO 30 HZ) ⇎

Thinking, Planning, Organising and Speaking

Let us start with beta brainwaves, because your brain is probably producing beta waves right now as you read this. In a state of beta, neurons fire rapidly. You can make connections quickly and easily and you are primed to do work that requires your full attention. It is probably your dominant waking consciousness, associated with being alert and concentrating.

Beta brainwaves help you to prepare for an exam, give a presentation, analyse and organise information, set and follow through on goals and carry out activities where mental alertness and high levels of concentration are key to success. Beta brainwaves also allow you to step back and witness your experience of life. This can help you temper and analyse emotions and be conscious in your responses.

A RANGE OF BETA

Beta brainwaves are divided into three bands according to their speed. High beta, close to the gamma end, reflects highly complex thought, moments of peak concentration and integrating new experiences. Middle beta is when we are actively engaged with a task or conversation, or figuring something out. Low Beta is connected to idle thinking or musing. Low Beta is closer to the alpha end, where you are in a relaxed, somewhat dreamy state. Research by Harvard scientists Matthew Killingsworth and Daniel Gilbert, published in 2010, found that we spend about 47 per cent of our awake time in a low beta state, with our minds wandering aimlessly or daydreaming about things completely unrelated to what we are doing. So our minds constantly mull over random details. One thought leads to another about what happened that day, what was said, what was seen, what was done, who we met and anything else we thought about. The unfortunate finding is that this idle daydreaming is also associated with depression and anxiety. So the conclusion of their study is that a wandering mind is an unhappy mind. This may be because a wandering mind tends to be a worrying mind, a distracted mind, a mind that struggles to switch off when we need rest, and that interferes with our ability to listen. It can make us more prone to addictive behaviour in an attempt to quiet our minds and artificially create inner peace. It also can compromise our health because it is not an energy efficient way to run the brain and body.

⇒ ALPHA BRAINWAVES (8 TO 12 HZ) ⇐

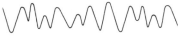

Gateway to the mindful zone

Alpha is a relaxed, peaceful state of mind. It is the resting state for the awake brain and can have a daydream-like and meditative quality to it. Completing a task and then sitting down to rest, taking a break from work and walking in the garden are all conducive to entering an alpha state. A light alpha state can also be achieved by taking a few deep breaths or time out to reflect. The alpha state is good for memory, and for consolidating things you have learned. Alpha brainwaves help you to feel calmly alert, which is a life skill that can be practised and improved upon. Having this skill can help you to keep calm in tough situations and to generally cope better with stress.

Ways to cultivate an alpha brainwave state include giving your thinking mind a break during the day, spending time in nature, balancing work, rest and play, physical exercise and using whatever relaxation methods work for you. Meditation, prayer and a good night's sleep are also alpha gateways. Cultivating alpha brainwave activity grows inner peace. The benefit of this is that those who find peace within also find it easier to live in peace with others.

EMOTIONAL STABILITY AND A SENSE OF WELLBEING
Higher alpha brainwave activity usually indicates a positive, stable and balanced emotional state. It allows you to be patient, grounded, calm and clear, which also gives you the space in your mind to notice your feelings and to respond in a more considered, rational way. The 'feel-good' effect of alpha brainwaves is associated with the release of bio-chemicals such as serotonin, which can help to counteract difficult emotions such as depression and anxiety. Alongside relaxation techniques some people may need to resolve unfinished emotional business that might stand in the way of true relaxation. Taking an emotional inventory and delving into challenging emotions in a supported way, might be necessary if you struggle to relax.

A RANGE OF ALPHA
Alpha ranges from daydreaming through to complete non-thinking. For example, you may still be thinking about, or reflecting on, your day, although with a dreamy quality to it. As you go deeper in alpha frequencies, closer to the theta end, your mind becomes rich with visual images associated with dreaming. The result is expanded awareness with access to intuition and deeper self-awareness. Both alpha and theta brainwaves

are great for creative thinking and problem solving. They give you a naturally creative state that you can apply to artistic endeavours and to everyday problem solving. Tuning in to alpha brainwaves can help you to see a current task in a new light, perhaps providing new insight and perspective.

⇒ THETA BRAINWAVES (4 TO 7 HZ) ⇐

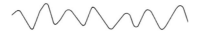

Emotional, imaginary realm

Theta brainwaves are present during deep relaxation and daydreaming as well as in meditation. Theta has been called a twilight state because of its fleeting appearance as you drift off to sleep and as you rise up out of deep sleep. It is also a twilight state because theta rests at the threshold of your subconscious mind. At these times it is like you are in a waking dream, receptive to imaginative ideas and creative thinking beyond your normal conscious awareness. It is great for 'out-of-the-box' thinking and is one reason for the saying 'sleep on it'. Essentially theta is an imagination wellspring.

Theta brainwaves are also produced when feeling emotional and they are involved in recording emotional memories. Because of this relationship between emotions, imagery and memory, focusing on any can give you access to all. For example, when we are feeling emotional theta stirs up associated imagery and memories. And this relationship can be used to our advantage when we apply visualisation to influence how we feel, and to work creatively with our memories.

Research shows that regular theta brainwave activity has great benefits, including boosting the immune system, enhancing creativity, and facilitating feelings of psychological wellbeing. Theta brainwaves can decrease mental fatigue and facilitate emotional processing.

DEEP THETA AT THE DELTA BORDER

The shamanic or spiritual trance state resides in the low theta brainwave frequency. Researcher Melinda Maxfield discovered that the steady, rhythmic beat of a drum, struck four-and-a-half times per second, is a shamanic tool for inducing the deepest part of the shamanic state of consciousness. Another example is the constant and rhythmic drone of Tibetan Buddhist chants that transports monks into realms of blissful meditation with brainwaves on the border of theta and delta. This frequency, together with delta brainwaves, is associated with the enlightened state as well as simply with a state of calm, clear and blissful inner peace. At these times there is deep, slow-wave resonance with nature giving a sense of interconnection or oneness with life, the universe and everything.

⇛ DELTA BRAINWAVES (0.1 TO 3 OR 4 HZ) ⇚

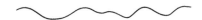

Deep dreamless sleep and restoration

Delta brainwaves are associated with deep, dreamless sleep. It is a time when your body and mind surrender all voluntary control, slipping into deep relaxation. It is a time when your body deeply restores and revives. Delta is the slowest of the five brainwave frequencies in which external awareness is suspended. In other words you generally have no conscious awareness while in a state of delta. For example, if you are woken from a deep sleep you can feel disorientated for a few moments as your consciousness catches up. Healing and regeneration are stimulated naturally in this state and various hormones, including human growth hormone (HGH), are released. This is why deep restorative sleep is so essential to health.

Delta frequencies, even while awake, regulate unconscious bodily processes such as the functioning of all of our body organs – heartbeat, breathing and digestion. There are many benefits associated with optimal delta wave functioning. These include getting a better night's sleep and boosting immune-system function. Deprivation of delta brainwaves can lead to feelings of depression, grogginess, feeling overwhelmed and generally feeling under the weather.

THE HIGHER PROPERTIES OF DELTA

Accessed while awake, delta and theta brainwaves, together, are found to enhance the capacity for intuition and empathy. This speaks to how quietude can wake both our sense of each other and our sense of the world, in a deeper way. An example of when this brainwave is produced is when parents emotionally attune to their infants. Delta brainwaves can also stimulate gamma brainwave frequencies as if the one spontaneously flips over into the other, such as when you are deeply absorbed in meditation or empathic rapport.

⇉ GAMMA BRAINWAVES (30 TO 200 HZ) ⇇

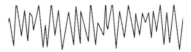

Super thinking and loving

Curiously, from our deepest state of relaxation, as well as from moments of total absorption and creative or physical flow, our brains can spontaneously flip over into a super-fast brainwave frequency called Gamma. Gamma brainwaves signify the highest state of perception and consciousness possible. In a gamma state the brain becomes more synchronised and cohesive, which allows for fast downloading, learning and processing of many aspects of information, all at once. This improves memory recall and perception. It also heightens sensory perception. Vision and hearing sharpen, and senses of smell, taste and touch are enhanced. Our brains become far more sensitive, noticing and picking up on far more information. This makes for a rich, sensory experience.

We all have gamma brainwave activity. It is the amount that varies. For example, gamma and theta brainwaves are present during the rapid eye movement (REM) stage of sleep. It is believed that this stage of sleep helps the brain to organise information into coherent images, thoughts and memories. Stress is found to decrease your brain's natural production of gamma brainwaves. As gamma brainwave activity decreases we become susceptible to depression, chronic stress and unfocused or impulsive thinking.

THE POWER OF LOVE

It is possible to generate gamma brainwave activity at will. Research has demonstrated that compassion is the key. For example, scientist Richard Davidson has demonstrated that when experienced Buddhist meditation practitioners meditate on compassion and loving kindness, their brainwaves go directly into gamma, averaging around 40 Hz. This experience has been associated with the 'feeling of blessings' as well as with feeling deeply content and blissful. In experienced meditators, studies have also shown an increase in brain activity in the part of the prefrontal cortex associated with self-control, compassion and empathy. Along with this increase is a reduction in the activity of the amygdala, to calm the fight or flight stress response. Gamma is a state of flow where you can feel connected with yourself in a deep, heartfelt way as well as feeling connected with others and the world. It is also a state that requires practice to achieve and maintain. As you would build fitness into your body, you can also build fitness into your heart and mind's ability to generate gamma frequencies. For a taste of this experience, and as a practice that can help you build this kind of fitness, take the Mindful Body Moment following this chapter.

SUPER GAMMA

Gamma brainwaves are also found to be the waves of heightened awareness and even psychic or out-of-body experiences. Extremely high brainwave frequencies above gamma have also been identified. They have been named hyper gamma or Lambda and Epsilon frequencies. The Epsilon state of consciousness is the state that advanced Yogis go into when they achieve suspended animation. These hyper gamma frequencies have also been associated with the ability of certain sects of Tibetan monks to meditate wearing only scant clothing, in freezing, sub-zero temperatures in the Himalayan mountains.

From a scientific perspective, gamma waves remain a mystery because they exist above the frequency of neuronal firing. It is speculated that gamma rhythms modulate perception and consciousness and that a greater presence of gamma relates to expanded consciousness and the mystical experience.

THE BRAINWAVES OF CHILDREN AND DEVELOPMENT INTO OLD AGE

In infants, theta and delta alternate as primary brainwave states. This can give babies an otherworldly quality as well as priming them for non-verbal, emotion-based connection and learning before they are able to verbalise and rationalise using the abilities that beta brainwaves will give them later in life. Adult females have been shown to have higher delta brainwave activity than males. This is true not just in humans but in most mammals. Perhaps this is nature at work, priming parents for attuning to their young as they synchronise with their babies to enhance bonding.

Young children mostly show a dominance of theta brainwave activity up until the age of six. This is associated with a rich imagination as well as with enhanced learning ability, making them sponges for absorbing new information. Around the age of six, alpha frequencies emerge and allow children to sit still in a classroom and to generally show more maturity. From the age of around twelve years beta brainwave activity increases and continues to develop into adulthood. This brings with it more maturity, and an ability to focus and engage with ever-higher levels of thinking. In some traditions age twelve is celebrated as a marker of entry into adulthood, which makes sense from this brainwave point of view. In the elderly, the dominant waking brainwave state is found to slow down to the alpha and theta range.

BALANCE, HEALTH AND THE PLACE FOR BODY AWARENESS

Optimum health is a state of consciousness that cycles between the five different brainwaves that balance and support each other. When your brain is in balance, there is an enhanced ability to fluidly and regularly transition between different brainwave frequencies, maximising your ability to think, learn, create and recall information. You are also more resilient to stress and can sleep deeply for much-needed restoration at the end of each day.

Some claim that there is an optimal biological frequency for health of mind and body that sits between alpha and theta, at 7.8 Hz. This is a healthy baseline to aspire towards and to cycle up and down from through the course of each day. It is not a static state to try and maintain.

Grounding and centring in your sensation-rich body is one way to achieve a baseline that is healthier and more energy efficient than living too much out of your thinking brain. One way to achieve this is to make your body the touchstone for your experience of life by referring to it at least as often as you refer to your thoughts. As the chapters of this book unfold, so will your understanding of how to apply body awareness to support a balanced, healthy life.

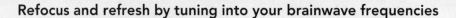

⇒ MINDFUL BODY MOMENT ⇐

Refocus and refresh by tuning into your brainwave frequencies

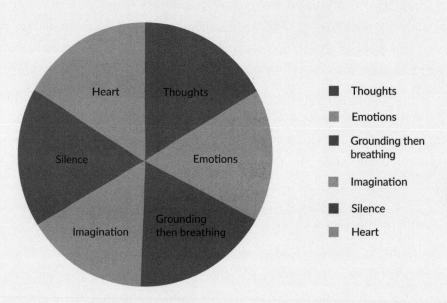

In the course of the day it is common for our concentration to get tangled up in our thoughts, feelings, body sensations and the many tasks at hand. Without being aware of it, this undifferentiated mix of mental, emotional and sensory input can be draining and can affect our clarity and precision. By consciously tuning in to the different brainwave frequencies, we can refresh our focus and take charge of where and how we direct our attention. By acknowledging and separating the different aspects of our internal experience, we can become more conscious and mindful about how we direct our attention thereafter. In this state we are invited to take a moment to acknowledge our internal reality and connect with a few moments of heartfelt care, which we can extend to ourselves and others.

This Mindful Body Moment involves moving attention to briefly notice different aspects of our internal experience, which will be associated with the different brainwave frequencies. You will be invited to notice thoughts, emotions and possibilities for feeling relaxed, and then be even more deeply relaxed. Attention is used like a flashlight, to shine light on these different aspects of internal experience and to finally come to rest in a refreshed state of mind-body being. Doing so can give you access to your brain's prefrontal cortex associated with mature, heartfelt behaviour. This can help your mental clarity as well as your creativity and adaptability.

Allow about 10 minutes to explore this for the first time; after that you can use it as a short break for a few minutes anytime and anywhere during your day. You can practise this Moment with your eyes open or closed, depending on your preference.

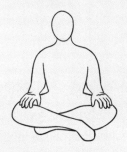

To start

Find a comfortable sitting position. Or you can be standing (especially once you know what to do and might choose to use this Moment when you are out and about). Because the thinking, beta brainwaves are where we spend most of our waking time, let's start from this point.

Notice thoughts

Begin by turning your attention to your thoughts, associated with the beta brainwave frequency. Spend a few moments with the contents of your thinking, simply being aware of them. No need to change what you find. Simply notice.

Notice emotions

Now turn your attention to your emotions, which indicate connection with the theta brainwave frequency (although not as deeply as your dreamy imagination that you will focus on in a moment). What feelings are with you now? Without needing to get into related stories, explore the possibility of simply being with your feelings, noticing where they live in your body and how they move inside you. No need to change what you find. Simply notice.

Notice body supported by the ground and room

Now turn your attention to your body. Feel the ground beneath your feet or, if you are sitting, feel the chair beneath you. Position both feet flat on the ground. If you are sitting, sit evenly on both hips to encourage feeling centred and balanced. Feel the solid support your body receives from the ground or your seat. You can also take a moment to imagine that the room or space you are in holds and contains you inside its walls, or that the nature surrounding you offers supportive holding or a sense of containment. Then take a moment to look around and take in your surroundings through fresh eyes. This grounding and sense of being held in the space that you are in can be an effective way to get your mind out of your thoughts and feelings and to help you move into more relaxed alpha, and eventually, delta brainwave frequencies.

Notice breathing

Now move your focus to your breathing. No need to change what you find. Simply notice your natural breathing for a few moments. Notice how your breathing enters and leaves your nose. If your mouth is open you might notice the movement of breath through your mouth too. Are you able to observe breathing rising and falling, filling and emptying other parts of your body too, such as your torso, or even your body as a whole? Allow your breathing to nourish, ventilate, ease and subtly energise you for these few moments while you are focusing on it. With this focus you can easily slip into alpha brainwave frequencies.

Notice imagination

As if you were about to fall asleep, invite your mind to drift into a half-awake, half-asleep dreamy state for a few moments. Go with the flow of what arises naturally and follow this for a few moments, noticing the images and body feelings associated with what appears from your imagination. Let any images come to you – you might think of film images to spark your imagination. Or you might remember an image from a recent dream and call it to mind now. Another way to invite images is to remember a time you felt emotional recently and then observe the images that flow from there. This is your theta brainwave bandwidth receiving your attention.

Notice absolute silence

Now imagine you are deeply asleep entering a place of complete stillness and quiet. There are no thoughts, no feelings, no movement in your imagination, or any awareness of your body. There is only quiet, and perhaps a sense of expansiveness or spaciousness associated with the delta brainwave frequency. Spend a few moments doing your best to stay connected with this deeply quiet space.

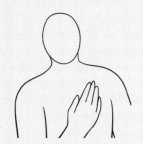

Hand on heart

Now place your right hand on your heart. Spend a few moments noticing and taking in what this action brings to your body and being. While holding your hand on your heart, return attention to your breathing, allowing your breathing to be natural and full and to ventilate your heartfelt moment. Call to mind someone or something you love. Maybe it is a child or a person in your life, a pet or your favourite place in nature. Whoever or whatever it is for you, spend a few moments holding this in mind to amplify your heart feelings. From there, simply soak up the experience for a few moments, allowing it to fill you and feed you. If it feels right for you today, you can radiate this love outwards to imagine touching someone or some group of people in your life. Perhaps you could extend this love even further out into the world as a warm gesture or wish of goodwill. Stay with this experience for as long as feels good and right. This can give you a sense of the warm glow associated with the gamma brainwave frequency.

Stretch and go

To close this Mindful Body Moment for now, take a deep breath and give your body a good stretch. Loosen up and bring some movement to your body, from head to toe. How do you feel now? Compare this sensation to how you felt at the start of the exploration. From this mindful body space, move on into the rest of your day.

CHAPTER 3

Change Your Posture, Change Your Mind

*Our bodies change our minds,
our minds can change our behavior
and our behavior can change our outcomes.*

AMY CUDDY

◆

Stating the obvious: When you feel down, your posture slumps and your head hangs low. Even if you fight it, when you are feeling low your impulse is to stoop your body in a downward direction. What might not be as obvious is that your posture can also perpetuate, or cause you to feel, a certain way and that changing your posture can change your mood and mind. Richard Petty, Professor of Psychology at Ohio State University, explains that the brain has areas that reflect feelings such as confidence, and when the specific area is triggered it is difficult to tell the difference between natural confidence and temporary confidence as a result of standing up straight. The brain responds in the same way to both. So your confidence can make you stand upright and standing upright can create confidence. The same applies to smiling. You can feel happy and smile naturally and you can smile to make you feel happier. Choosing to smile is seen to yield the same warm effects as smiling naturally, such as increasing 'feel-good' hormones like endorphins, serotonin and dopamine, reducing the stress hormone cortisol, increasing relaxation and increasing the sense of pleasure in doing a task.

Professor Erik Peper of San Francisco State University also refers to posture and confidence, adding to our understanding of how the body affects the mind, in this case relating to memories. He offers that in an upright position of confidence, it is easier to recall empowering and positive personal traits. On the other hand, a slouched position tends to bring up memories of feeling defeated in some way – hopeless, helpless and powerless. In other words, our thoughts and memories are dependent on how we feel at the time, which is influenced or reinforced by our posture.

⇒ BODY LANGUAGE IN ACTION ⇐

Try it out for yourself. First try smiling for its own sake, and track how your body responds. Stay with this awareness for a few moments and absorb the feelings. Then stand or sit in a slouched position and look downwards. How do you feel now, and what kinds of thoughts spring to mind? Notice this for a few moments. Finally, try standing or sitting in an upright position with your chest open and your chin up. How do you feel now, and what kinds of thoughts and memories arrive? Experimenting with your body in these ways can give you a sense of how changing your body can change your mind, your mood and your outlook. Different postures also change you physiologically, influencing things like muscle tension, quality of breathing, blood flow, heart rate and digestion, which all contribute to the shifts in how you feel.

This can raise questions about our modern lifestyles. Some of us sit for long hours at a desk in front of a computer screen and most of us look down to our smart phones many times every day. This can reinforce a slumped posture associated with reducing a person's energy levels (not to mention increasing a propensity towards headaches and neck and shoulder pains). With this in mind, Peper recommends looking away from your screen every now and then as well as hanging photos of people you love, slightly higher than eye level or above your desk, so that you have to look up to see them. You can also use reminders to sit upright such as on your computer or on post-it notes. Peper also recommends that when you experience negative thoughts, you should try not to carry them around with you, especially if you are also walking around in a slumping posture. Rather, write them down on a piece of paper and throw the paper in the bin. Taking some symbolic action to discard them may help to shift your focus to a more positive perspective.

IT ONLY TAKES TWO MINUTES

Harvard University researcher Amy Cuddy suggests that adopting 'high power' body positions for just two minutes a day significantly boosts testosterone levels and lowers cortisol levels. A 'high power' pose is an upright, open body position (such as standing with hands on hips and head held high like a superhero). A stance such as this is said to boost confidence and reduce stress or anxiety.

Two minutes is proposed as the optimal time for gaining the benefits from these positions. For example, in Erik Peper's studies he found that two minutes of skipping (in contrast to walking in a slouched position) significantly changes energy levels, effectively lifting your level of feel-good hormones. Discovering how quickly and easily we can influence how we feel and think, simply by changing our posture or moving differently, is empowering. We already know from the touch chapter that a single touch can instantaneously raise oxytocin levels with accompanying loving feelings, so if your posture includes conscious touch, such as with a hand to your heart, it need not even take two minutes to change your mood and mind in measurable ways.

⇒ BOOSTING QUALITIES YOU NEED ⇐

In this section are four postural signatures that can give you access to useful qualities. With these you can boost loving kindness, confidence, zest for life, and centred thoughtfulness, depending on what you might wish for at different times.

To familiarise yourself with the postures, copy the following pictures, trying each one in turn. Hold each position for a few seconds, really feeling how it affects you, before moving on to the next.

Because you are focusing on the upper body in each pose, you may either sit or stand. Notice which come naturally to you – which poses you relate to easily, and which you do not relate to easily. You might also remember times when you could access feeling a certain way even if right now it does not resonate with you. Simply notice what comes up for you when you try each pose.

You might get a sense of how each can associate with personality or distinct styles of being in the world. Each posture also has the potential to change how you feel and, with it, change your body's biochemistry too.

Dr Helen Fisher speaks about this connection between personality and bio-chemistry, in her book *Why Him? Why Her?*, which discusses attraction patterns in intimate adult relationships. Through her research, Dr Fisher found four ways that personality traits are reliably linked with bio-chemistry. This involves two hormones, estrogen and testosterone, and two neurotransmitters, dopamine and serotonin. Associated with the four postural signatures that you just tried out, hand on heart can be seen to represent estrogen qualities, hands on hips represents testosterone qualities, hands reaching up high represents dopamine qualities and the prayer pose represents serotonin qualities.

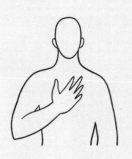

BOOSTING LOVING KINDNESS

Placing your hand on your heart awakens your skin to the power of touch, helping you to feel more connected with yourself and others. This posture conveys sincerity and caring and invites an introspective, feeling-focused mood. These qualities are associated with estrogen as well as with oxytocin, which works together with estrogen in the body. Both women and men have access to estrogen and its related qualities – such as nurturing.

Other ways to boost loving kindness:

Soften your eyes so they may give out warm, heartfelt energy.

Soak in a warm bath. Oxytocin levels rise in response to warmth.

Listen to soothing music – a study of patients recovering from open-heart surgery found that when they listened to soothing music, their oxytocin levels increased. As a result they were less stressed and this had a positive influence on their healing.

Practise random acts of kindness. Research shows that even if the recipient is not aware of your kindness, your oxytocin levels rise because of how satisfied you can feel.

Write or share a few things that you are grateful for each day.

HORMONES AND PERSONALITY

Dr Fisher describes estrogen-dominant personality types as Negotiators. Traits include being unassuming, agreeable and supportive. Negotiators have many strong social connections. They are naturally empathic, nurturing, trusting and introspective and seek meaning and identity. Other ways Dr Fisher describes Negotiators are that they are: idealistic and able to see the big picture; good philosophers drawing on web-thinking abilities; have a tendency to be reflective, intuitive and compassionate; are imaginative, especially in synthesising and organising the ideas of others in novel ways (as opposed to the innovatively creative, out-of-the-box thinking of dopamine-related traits).

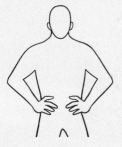

BOOSTING CONFIDENCE

If you need a confidence and assertiveness boost, or you wish to calm anxiety and reduce shyness, use a 'high power' pose for two minutes (as Cuddy's research encourages). Cuddy and her team classified different body positions as 'high power' or 'low power' poses based on their effects. In general, the 'high power' poses are open across the chest area and upright. Examples are, standing with your hands on your hips (think of Superman or Wonder Woman) or either sitting or standing with hands behind your neck and elbows open so that your chest and shoulders are open. These body positions allow you to inflate your chest area, displaying confidence. Like an elephant fanning out its ears, these poses make you look and feel bigger. The contrast is 'low power' poses. These are closed body positions, closed in around your chest area, such as holding your arms crossed, and slouching with head downwards.

While holding the 'high power' pose, take a few conscious breaths, perhaps breathing in for a count of three and out for a count of five, to encourage your body to relax into this confident pose. Even if this feels unnatural for you, knowing that you can increase your confidence when you need to is empowering. It can help give you a boost before an important presentation, an interview, a challenging meeting, or anytime you feel you need confidence.

As a personality type, Dr Fisher describes this kind of person as a Director. Traits include a tendency to be highly analytical, competitive and emotionally contained while focused on grand achievement out in the world. They tend to be extroverted and task-focused, independent achievers and can have a heroic side. Other words to describe them are assertive, or aggressive at times, and single-minded; they are systemic thinkers with an interest in underlying rules and patterns; direct, decisive and easily able to speak their minds. These people are biologically primed to be more assertive, confident, less reactive to stress and able to handle pressure situations well. Dr Fisher also refers to them as finger pointers!

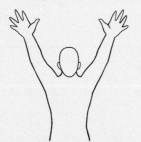

BOOSTING ZEST FOR LIFE

Standing with hands reaching up to the sky can give you a feeling of being full of life or extending to experience life to the full. It is a pose an athlete may do without even thinking, as they victoriously cross the finish line, or how you may react when reaching the top of a mountain or accomplishing something significant. The victory pose has been identified as a 'high power' pose associated with testosterone, but it has a more excitable, elevated feel to it than the rooted strength of the confidence-boosting pose with hands on hips. This excitability is a quality associated with the neurotransmitter dopamine, which works closely with testosterone i.e. when testosterone levels are high the brain's release of dopamine is stimulated; when testosterone is low dopamine is inhibited. Both are associated with extroversion in different ways. The hands-on-hips pose has a more determined 'I am the boss', task-focused feel to it, whereas the victory pose has more of a soaring 'I did it', emotion-focused feel to it. Other qualities associated with dopamine include excitement, adventurousness, risk-taking and a fun-loving attitude.

Dopamine has been nicknamed our 'motivation molecule', giving a rush of 'I can do it!' and 'I did it' feelings. This is because of the key role that it plays in our pleasure-reward system. Richard Depue, an expert in the neurobiology of personality, emotion and temperament, has found a connection between dopamine and responsiveness to incentives and rewards. The greater the brain's responsiveness to dopamine, the more likely a person is to experience what Depue calls 'positive emotionality'. This includes feeling excited and eager, or even elated, when going after goals and anticipating rewards. This goal-reward state feels good and motivates us to move towards achieving what we want. But if you don't get what you are after then dopamine levels can drop, which is not a good feeling. Not enough dopamine can leave you with little energy, struggling to concentrate and feeling unmotivated, apathetic, lethargic and possibly depressed. At these times you may turn to self-destructive, addictive behaviours for an artificial dopamine boost.

We are not designed to experience a non-stop dopamine high, however. But because surges of dopamine are so pleasurable, some of us can fall prey to the instant gratification of addictive behaviour in the chase after the dopamine rush. This of course is not sustainable. Luckily there are healthy ways to boost dopamine-related qualities. To follow are some ideas for how to do so.

Healthy ways to boost zest for life

Try new things and wake your sense of adventure.

Accomplish small things and give yourself small wins each day. Dopamine increases when you finish tasks no matter how small. Finishing the washing, spring cleaning or getting to the bottom of your to-do list – completing anything can give you that 'I did it' satisfaction associated with dopamine. For the big things you want to achieve, break them down into small, achievable steps.

Tap into your creativity in whatever ways work for you.

Listen to music. Studies have shown that listening to music causes your brain to release dopamine. Even playing a tune in your mind can cause your dopamine levels to rise.

Exercise + novelty. Exercise releases 'feel good' chemicals like serotonin, endorphins, and dopamine. Even light exercise, such as taking the dog out for a walk, a gentle Yoga class, or playing in the waves at the beach, can do the trick. Adding novelty, like running a new route or trying something new while exercising, gives even more of a dopamine boost – in the same way that competitive sport and even playing with your children, in fun and active ways, can also do.

Meditate or pray to see life more clearly through fresh eyes.

As a personality type, Dr Fisher refers to this kind of person as an Explorer. Her views on this as a personality type include being adventurous, novelty and sensation seeking, unusually creative and curious. She adds that they are spontaneous and impulsive, ever optimistic, irreverent, autonomous and love to have fun! These people tend to be curious, energetic and flexible in their choices, and tend not to be particularly introspective. They can have an excellent attention span but only when inspired and engaged in activities towards achieving rewarding goals. When motivated, they can be visionaries and truly innovative thinkers. But the minute they lose interest they can get bored, restless and unable to focus.

BOOSTING CENTRED THOUGHTFULNESS

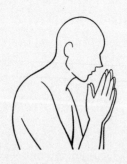

Actions like placing your index finger on your chin or temple or resting your chin on your fist reflectively as in the thinker pose, can have the effect of turning your attention inwards into your thoughts. The prayer pose yields a similar effect, differing by perhaps evoking more of a quiet, contemplative quality than the thinker pose. The prayer pose has also been linked with feeling centred, contemplative and content. The bio-chemical associated with feeling this way is serotonin. Serotonin is a neurotransmitter manufactured in the brain and in the intestines. There is a close relationship between serotonin and estrogen, with estrogen necessary for the production of serotonin. Psychologically, serotonin and estrogen can be linked to introspection. Both can stabilise mood.

Low levels of serotonin have been linked with psychological challenges including depression, obsessive-compulsive disorder, anxiety, panic, attention deficit disorders, impulse control disorders and excessive anger. Abundant serotonin is associated with a quiet and deep sense of contentment and wellbeing. This is in contrast with dopamine, which also contributes to our happiness, but differently. Dopamine is the excited, inspired state of happiness. Serotonin is the quiet, deep sense of happiness. They can be experienced by the same person at different times. Sometimes we might prefer novel, thrilling, and sensation-seeking dopamine-related qualities. Other times we might prefer the quieter, serotonin-related qualities such as the warm glow of happiness felt from the inside out.

The prayer pose is one easy way to boost qualities associated with serotonin. It can quickly awaken a contemplative mindset and help you consult with a higher source of wisdom than perhaps your usual thinking allows. Similarly, meditation and prayer can cultivate internal poise as you connect with your contemplative nature in a spiritual way. Below are some other ideas for boosting qualities associated with serotonin.

Mood management:

Feeling happy has been positively correlated with the brain's synthesis of serotonin, whereas feeling sad has been negatively correlated. So the more you invest in your happiness, the higher your serotonin levels will be. For you that may include living a meaningful life, being healthy, having healthy relationships and good social networks. So, what makes you happy? Or, what is standing in the way of your happiness? These are good questions to ask yourself when you are feeling down, and may encourage you to seek any support you might need to get there.

Exposure to sunlight:

A minimum of 30 minutes exposure to bright, natural light per day can stimulate feel-good bio-chemicals including serotonin. Substitute sunlight, such as the Scandinavian idea of a 'Light Cafe', for times of the year when sunlight is limited, can also be effective.

Exercise:

Exercise is known to improve mood and raise serotonin levels. Regular exercise can help to keep depression, anxiety and general negativity at bay.

Eat healthily:

Because serotonin is largely produced in the gut, eating healthily helps promote healthy serotonin levels.

Meditation:

Meditation helps you to improve focus and concentration. It also grows your internal witness to help you see life more clearly, while enhancing your access to intelligent, rational thinking and inner wisdom when you need some guidance.

Monitor your self-talk:

If you had a friend who spoke to you as you sometimes speak to yourself, would you keep this friend? Pause now and again, especially if you are feeling anxious or stressed, and listen to your self-talk. Is it constructive or destructive? How can you change your mental chatter to be more supportive and motivating? Try saying something new to yourself and notice how that affects you.

Think and write:

If you wish to develop your ability to be more analytical and thoughtful, you could keep a journal, which might reflect on your experiences for a period of time. Or you could write down your goals, dreams or plans for the future and then identify long- and short-term goals towards achieving them. You could take pen to paper to consider any problem in detail, such as considering the pros and cons, different solutions, or creative ideas towards crafting a practical plan.

As a personality type, Dr Fisher refers to this kind of person as a Builder. She characterises them as cautious, conventional, loyal, conscientious and tactful, as well as feeling a sense of duty and having respect for authority figures. She adds that they are calm and self-contained. This kind of person can display self-confidence but only when they feel well prepared. They have a need for schedules, order and plans, and can make good managers. Of all the personality styles, this one is the most able to feel quietly content in their own company. They tend to be introverted and quietly task focused, as opposed to focused on emotions in themselves and others.

WE ARE ALL A MIX OF TRAITS

With awareness we can all recognise how some personality traits come naturally to us. For some of us one style screams out as true. For others, two or sometimes three personality traits resonate. Like a paint palette, we all have all the personality shades available to us, just like we all have the full range of bio-chemicals present in our brains and bodies. They do not live in isolation inside of us; they all affect each other and work together with many other chemicals and systems in the body and brain. It is the ratio of one to another that can distinguish us, uniquely colouring each of our ways of being in the world. So looking at them as four distinct styles, although that does not convey the complexity of how our bio-chemistry works, is still useful and can feel true. It can offer us a useful lens for understanding ourselves and each other. It is important to note that there is no 'best' personality style; they are all just different. Each has strengths and areas of challenge. It can also be empowering to discover that even though we naturally lean towards particular styles of being in the world, it is possible to acquire traits of different personality styles that we might wish to lean into at different times.

REFLECTION

» Which of the four postures and associated traits do you relate to most naturally?

» Can you recognise traits of others in your life that might be the same or different to yours?

» Which personality traits are your least developed?

» How does this affect you?

» How does this play out in your relationships at home and work?

⇾ NATURE OR NURTURE? ⇽

Are we born with a personality type or are our personalities shaped by our families, communities and environment? The answer is probably both. There are certain things that we are born with that are enduring, including aspects of our bio-chemistry that shape our inherent personality. Upbringing and life experience also play a part in shaping us, changing aspects of our personality and behaviour as we move through life. Some of us are even able to override our biology to think and behave in ways that are not innate, through exposure to, for example, family and friends and adaptation to our environment. Arguably we may never feel quite at home in our own skin if we have made a drastic shift from who we innately are. Practising boosting our different personality traits is a valuable life skill, which can help us to grow personally and improve our relationships with the different kinds of people around us.

LIVING A BALANCED AND FULFILLING LIFE

If you are too strong in one personality style and underdeveloped in another, you can feel out of balance or unable to achieve what you wish for in life. To live a balanced, fulfilled life, no matter what your natural tendencies are, you can benefit from drawing on various qualities at different times. Perhaps your great striving has led to a lack of inner peace or to a lack of connection with your loved ones. Perhaps your serenity or contentment has led to a lack of motivation for taking your work out into the world. Or perhaps in working with others, or in your leadership, you realise you may need to be more patient or learn to assert yourself more effectively. These are traits that you can deliberately boost when you need them, by using your posture as a proactive reminder.

There are also stages of life that might lend themselves to different traits. For example, when we start out on a career path or in a new job we may need extra courage and personal reach as we encounter new territories and stretch our abilities. Or when we start a family we may be drawn to a quieter, more introspective lifestyle as we become enchanted and perhaps exhausted by the new children in our lives. And at any time of life we might find ourselves bored of the old routine and wishing to muster up the enthusiasm and courage to explore something new.

TRAITS FOR TEAMS

Referring to personality traits can also apply to teams or any systems that require a variety of traits to function optimally. For example, a team without courage, strong action or vision, may stagnate. A team that does not care for each other may lose good talent when the team environment becomes cold and hostile. A team without sufficient analysis, assessment and reflection could rush into changes and actions and repeatedly make mistakes that could have been avoided. A balanced team needs access to all personality traits in order to be able to see gaps and achieve its greatest results.

Applied to leadership, a good leader ideally knows their strengths and areas of limitation, and is able to adapt to different types of people and manage diversity in the groups they work with. A good leader is also able to access the personality style appropriate for the situation, such as drawing on bold, single-mindedness to make a final or quick decision, or drawing on consultation to make sure different voices are included. Martin Luther King Jr. powerfully encapsulates the interplay of different personality attributes in this excerpt from his speech in 1967: 'What is needed is a realisation that power without love is reckless and abusive, and love without power is sentimental and anemic. Power at its best is love implementing the demands of justice, and justice at its best is power correcting everything that stands against love.' This is leadership at its best.

⇁ MINDFUL BODY REFLECTION ⇀

Moving closer to the truth

In truth, our personalities and our lives are not fixed. Even if we associate with being confident or nurturing or inspiring or contemplative, at times we might behave differently depending on our circumstances. When we turn our attention inwards to our bodies, we can come to notice how we are constantly in motion, never static, and never just one way in life. We might behave differently at work to the way we behave with our families. We might have a happy persona and a stressed-out one. In one context we might feel shy, but in another we have access to feeling confident. Or, if we often feel confident, we might notice some shame or humility creeping in at times, too. We are, in truth, a fluid soup of feelings that change in response to our experiences of life.

As we turn our attention to sensations in our bodies we can come to know our bodies from the inside out, as three-dimensional and as vitally alive. The very act of bringing attention to the body – perhaps by noticing how we are standing and beginning to play with posture and quality of movement – can change how we feel. For example, the simple act of looking inwards can wake our calming parasympathetic nervous system to naturally start a process of relaxation which can be helpful at times of stress. When stressed, our natural instinct is to fix attention on our problems or on feeling threatened, as if in survival mode. But if we resist and turn our attention inwards to notice our body instead of our thoughts, it can remind us that we can take charge of our body's reactions. Perhaps we notice that our shoulders are drawn up, or our jaw and eyes are tense, or our breath is held. Then we might take a few deep breaths, release areas of tension and adjust our posture to feel more comfortable, empowered or uplifted (by using some of the ideas presented in this book). The key is self-awareness. So as you go about your days, begin to experiment with your posture, noticing how this might shift your state of mind, emotions and outlook.

⇒ MINDFUL BODY PROCESS ⇐

Strengthening adaptability and resilience from body to mind

This Mindful Body Process invites you to catch yourself in a negative state such as shame, anxiety, depression, irritation or annoyance. You are then invited to pause and notice your body's posture and then contrast it with a positive and helpful state. If you are not actually bothered in this moment, then remember a time when you might have felt this way so that you can try out the practice. Once you know what to do, you can use it on the spot anytime you catch yourself in a negative state that you can shift to become more positive.

You are invited to hold, alternate and experience the contrast of each posture long enough for your brain and body to really register the experience. This juxtaposing of positive and negative can support the brain's neuroplasticity. This is especially true when we make a habit of challenging old, self-limiting habits, replacing them with new, helpful habits.

To start with:

Catch yourself when you are feeling emotionally bothered (or think of a time you might have felt this way – perhaps a time you felt hurt, ashamed, irritated, full of rage or perhaps defeated, helpless or hopeless. Spend a few moments remembering this feeling and what triggered you to feel this way. As you do so, notice how your feelings live in your body and allow your posture to shape around it. When you find a position that feels like a true representation of your state of mind and emotions, hold the position for about 30 seconds so that your brain and body can really notice the experience.

Then invite your body, not your mind, to find an opposite or contrasting posture, one that feels different and helpful compared with how you just were. Follow your body for a few moments as you open to where your body wants to lead you, breathing and feeling into a new possibility. When you find what feels like a satisfying new position as counterpoint to the first posture, hold this position for about 30 seconds, which will allow the experience to permeate your body, your bio-chemistry and your mind.

From there you are invited to play with contrasting the positive and negative postures a few times before settling into the positive. Once you are clear about your negative and positive postures, move from one posture to the other a few times, spending a few moments, perhaps ten seconds or so at a time, holding each posture. You can also explore a fluid process of moving between the postures, in your own way, to feel into their contrast. For some it might be feeling restless and tight, turning into feeling free. For others it might be feeling slumped and heavy, shifting to feeling lighter and more willing to move; or feeling frozen, easing into more breathing space and flow. There is no right or wrong, only what feels true and helpful for you. To end, move into the positive posture.

To close this exploration for now, spend a few moments, perhaps another 30 seconds, in the positive posture. You might breathe and move a bit to explore this new terrain and to settle into it as you notice the effects on your body, emotions and mind. From this space, if you wish, you can ask your positive self for some advice related to a current situation. Then be open to a response in thought, feeling or image as you perhaps open to fresh ideas.

⇥ MINDFUL BODY MOMENT ⇤

Reminding yourself of a positive state

Following the Mindful Body Process of juxtaposing a negative with a positive body-mind state, your positive state gives you a ready Mindful Body Moment to take forwards for use on the spot, anytime and anywhere. It is helpful to spend a few moments each day, during the days that follow, to recall and take on the posture and mindset of your new way of being, so as to anchor it in your body, brain and behaviour.

The more often you use exercises like this to respond to challenging feelings, the more ingrained your response flexibility can become in general. This can build your emotional resilience as you realise you have the ability to change your posture to change your mind.

CHAPTER 4

Stress and Body First-Aid

It's not the load that breaks you down, it's the way you carry it.

LOU HOLTZ

⇉ DIFFERENT TYPES OF STRESS ⇇

Stress management is not 'one size fits all'. Stress can take on many forms and can require different interventions. Stress can be triggered by daily pressures and demands, which can be experienced as acute, transient stress. Some people are more prone to stress than others, depending on their work and life situation. Stress can sometimes be linked to socio-economic or political factors, too. When stress is experienced on a regular basis over a period of time, it can leave a stress residue in your body and mind so that you never really feel free of it. This can lead to a chronic condition, sometimes stemming back to early childhood emotional wounds or to traumatic experiences. Some ways that this can manifest is in conditions such as clinical depression or anxiety together with hyper-sensitivity, hyper-vigilance and heightened reactivity to the otherwise manageable occurrence of daily stress.

Acute, transient stress in small amounts can be motivating and exciting. Although too much too often can push us over the edge towards lingering, chronic stress that can deplete our energy, distract our ability to focus and affect our health.

Causes of stress can include time pressures, lack of good-quality sleep, parenting challenges, relationship stress, work stress, emotional or psychological stress resulting from short- or long-term disappointments, needs not met, loss and other emotional triggers. There is also anticipatory stress – when we fear something in our future and question our ability to overcome it – and situational stress or trauma when we might be taken by surprise by sudden incidents that we might not feel able to cope with. These are just a few of the possible causes of stress that we may experience.

STRESS RELIEF

For stress relief there are general, helpful strategies applicable to anyone and specific strategies that target different kinds of stress. For acute stress that appears in short bursts, applying general stress-management strategies, such as taking deep breaths, going for a walk, talking through an argument, or using self-supportive touch, can usually be applied fairly easily and effectively. It is when stress becomes chronic that it can push us too far so that we hold more stress than our bodies and minds can handle. At these times we might feel unable to regulate our stress with simple strategies such as those mentioned above. Or perhaps these strategies provide only short moments of relief, which is insufficient. In the case of chronic stress, professional or community support might be needed to gradually address the past and to assist in building coping strategies towards improving emotional resilience and a sense of wellbeing.

With the skill of body mindfulness it is possible to improve our ability to bounce back from adversity. It can also help us maintain a less reactive, more resilient and adaptable way of being. This skill is associated with the development of a part of the brain called the prefrontal cortex. Let's pause to introduce the brain in a basic way so as to understand the role of the prefrontal cortex and how to encourage its development.

⇛ THREE BRAIN REGIONS: THREE WAYS TO EXPERIENCE LIFE ⇚

In the 1970s, neurologist Paul MacLean proposed that we have not one, but three brains. His Triune Brain Theory proposes that each part of the brain evolved over time, one by one, until there were three distinct yet interconnected brains. According to MacLean each of these brains has its own special intelligence, its own subjectivity, its own sense of time and space and its own memory. They affect each other and work together and they are distinct, each with its own purpose and function.

These three parts of the brain, from bottom to top, are the reptilian or 'low' brain, which is the least evolved part of the brain, the mammalian or 'mid' brain, and the neo-mammalian or 'high' brain, which is the most evolved part of the brain and the home of the prefrontal cortex. These different brain regions associate with different aspects of our human nature. Bringing awareness to each is a life skill that can be helpful.

Although The Triune Brain model has been criticised by scientists who believe the model is overly simplistic, it remains useful for showing how and why logic and reason can break down when emotions and stress run high. The theory also points to ideas for what to do about stress.

REPTILIAN BRAIN AND YOUR BODY SELF

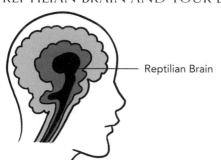

Reptilian Brain

The reptilian brain is the oldest part of the brain and the first of our three brains to evolve. It includes the brainstem and the cerebellum. It is the dominant brain in reptiles, hence the name 'reptilian brain'. It does not require conscious thinking; instead it concerns itself with instinctual activities, survival and reproduction. It commands our freeze, startle or shock response and works together with the mammalian brain in the fight or flight response to threat. Both the 'low' and 'mid' brain regions are relied upon to keep us safe by responding quicker than thinking. The reptilian brain also keeps basic body functions going without conscious intervention, such as controlling balance, breathing, the beating of our hearts, digestion and cycles of feeling awake and tired. Added to this are physical abilities that become automatic once mastered, such as walking, riding a bicycle and anything that we practise for long enough so that it feels like it comes naturally.

You can think of the reptilian brain as governing your body self. It can feel like the dancer or the athlete in you, or simply the animal body that carries you through life in your particular style. It occupies itself with actions like eating, sleeping, mating and defending, as well as sensing, moving, scanning and adapting. With self-observation, which is a function of the 'high' mammalian brain, you can become curious about living more consciously in your body, such as feeling into your body's natural style of moving and engaging with the world through your senses.

When you feel in any way threatened, your body reacts first. Before you have a chance to think about it, your eyes, facial expression and posture have shifted in preparation for attack, defence or escape. Research shows that your brain and body have prepared or organised for movement, like picking up a glass of water, seconds before you are even aware of your desire to pick up the glass. So your body receives and transmits intentions and messages moments before your conscious thinking mind becomes aware of it. Because of this quick reacting, micro-expressions in your face such as a quick lift of your eyebrows, in surprise, or a jutting forward of your jaw, in anger, or the dilation of your pupils, can give away your honest reactions to someone curious enough to pay close attention. Humans are designed to pick up facial cues in others to help make a quick assessment whether they are friend or foe. Then our thinking catches up to try to understand or override what is going on.

The reptilian brain primarily generates delta brainwaves, the slow waves of deep, dreamless sleep. When you are feeling safe this state results in you feeling naturally relaxed and with a clear mind. Look into the eyes of a relaxed baby or the eyes of a lizard and you can get a sense of this. It is the feeling of nowhere to go, nothing to do, just to be here now.

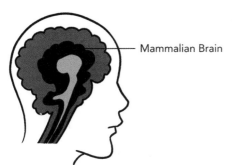

Mammalian Brain

MAMMALIAN BRAIN AND YOUR EMOTIONAL SELF

Moving up the evolutionary scale is the mammalian brain. MacLean coined the term 'limbic system' to characterise this mammalian portion of our brains. You can think of this portion of the brain as governing your emotional self. It is the part of your brain that responds emotionally to life and it stores emotion-rich memory. Theta brainwaves dominate the functioning of this portion of the brain. These are the brainwaves of imagination and they go hand in hand with our experience of emotions and memory.

This part of the brain is like social glue, binding us together and letting us know how our relationships affect us. Think of playful dolphin families, the affection of a mother lioness towards her cubs, the attentive grooming behaviour of monkeys, or elephants mourning their dead – these are all examples of the sociality of mammals. The mammalian brain compels parents to nurture and care for their offspring, with tenderness and warmth. It also creates complex emotional bonds and a sense of kinship in social groups, as well as the ability to read emotional states, predict them and respond to the likely behaviour of others in a group. The longing to belong is also born in this part of the brain.

Everything according to this emotional part of the brain is categorised into agreeable or disagreeable, guiding us to move towards pleasure and avoid pain. It is an impulsive, powerful and very influential part of the brain, which adds pleasure or displeasure to the reptilian brain's natural survival instincts.

The fight or flight response is generated by the amygdala, which lives inside the mammalian brain and engages the reptilian brain to physically carry out its commands. There is also another threat response called 'tend and befriend', which serves a limbic, socially binding kind of function. Dr Shelley Taylor and her research team put forward this model, proposing that 'tend and befriend' is an alternative instinctual stress response that some people naturally gravitate towards. It is usually associated with women, although men can also draw on it. The association with women has primitive roots. In primitive terms, males would usually defend and protect the perimeters of a group, tending towards the fight or flight response. Females, on the other hand, could have an equally strong instinct to tend to their loved ones and to pull together in the community for the sake of mutual defence and preservation.

There are two other 'brains' associated with your emotional brain. One is located in your heart and one in your gut area. The heart 'brain' was introduced by Dr J. Andrew Armour in 1991. He pointed out that the heart also contains neurons that actively communicate with the amygdala, providing an integral part of the emotional limbic system. This can explain the connection between the heart and emotions. It is also perhaps why placing a hand on your heart area can cause such a noticeable shift to your emotional and brain state. The gut or enteric 'brain', discovered in 1998 by Dr Michael Gershon, has also been found to communicate directly with the amygdala, also connecting your gut to your emotions and stress. If you are ever struggling to connect with your emotions, pay attention to your heart and gut areas, perhaps breathe into these areas or place a hand on each (one on your heart, one on your gut) so that you can connect with your feelings more easily.

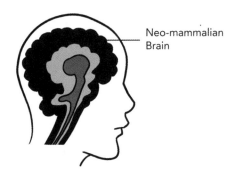
Neo-mammalian Brain

NEO-MAMMALIAN BRAIN AND YOUR THINKING SELF

This most highly evolved portion of the brain is referred to by different names including the 'neocortex' and the 'neo-mammalian' brain. It is the rational or reasoning part of the brain that is home to the prefrontal cortex. Paul MacLean refers to this part of the brain as the mother of invention, and the father of abstract thought.

Think of this 'brain' as your rational or thinking self. In brainwave terms it produces anything from relaxed, reflective alpha- to busy beta brainwaves. It offers you the ability to analyse, assess, plan, organise, figure out and reflect on life. It helps you to step out of the intensity of emotional and physical experience to observe, attempt to make sense of, and comment on life. Here you can meet your human abilities to be creative, to have feelings about your feelings, to debate morality, philosophise and put emotions and instant gratification aside as you embark on a journey towards long-term goals, such as education and professional achievement. This is also the part of the brain that allows you to be mindful, bringing conscious attention and intention to how you respond to life.

Our ability to think also expands our emotional palette as new shades of emotion evolve from thoughts about our feelings and being able to be aware of, and hold, a mix of these feelings. We can also have thoughts that inspire positivity or negativity and we can use language to motivate ourselves and each other.

This part of the brain interacts with the lower brain regions by collecting data from the lower brain, sifting and analysing what it finds and making decisions based on its assessment of these findings. It can also become an integrative function of all brain regions, especially when functioning optimally. Unlike the reptilian and mammalian brains, the neo-mammalian brain offers the bigger picture. This bigger picture comes from the ability to think beyond the present moment as well as to string basic information together to form more complex understandings or theories. In our daily lives it is what helps us to function and interact calmly, coherently and effectively. It is available to us when we feel in control and able to balance many aspects of our lives and responsibilities.

When functioning well, this part of the brain, and particularly the prefrontal cortex, can be summarised as wise, attuned and empathic. It can help us carry out daily tasks and move towards goals with intelligence, intention and mindfulness. It is also relationship-oriented and is shaped in our early relationships. This influences our capacity to tune in to ourselves and others, to empathise, and to regulate our emotions. Later in the book we will explore this early influence more deeply.

Along with intelligence and empathic attunement, the prefrontal cortex also serves a cohesive role in the brain, integrating the communication between, and synchronising, the functioning of the brain as a whole. When functioning optimally, we can experience frequent mental clarity, inspiration, insight and sense of flow. When activated optimally, the prefrontal cortex can generate moments of gamma brainwave activity, which sweep across the brain, from front to back, around 40 times per second. This sweeping stimulates many brain areas. On brain-scan images this can be seen as many areas of the brain lighting up at once as electrical activity and energy patterns in the brain become more widespread. This type of synchronisation can appear in the brain at times of intense creativity as well as times of deep absorption, such as in empathic rapport and compassion-based meditation.

Other benefits of a well-developed prefrontal cortex include a strong ability to regulate the nervous system. This can calm our stress responses and make us more emotionally resilient. A well-developed prefrontal cortex also hones our morality by aligning us with the bigger picture and allowing us the capacity for compassion.

EMOTIONAL FLOODING AND FEELING OUT OF CONTROL

Although we are capable of reason, emotional control, and behaving in a calm and loving way, we don't operate like this all the time, especially when visited by life's little or grand annoyances. In a moment, we can be set off on a rampage, losing our temper, or falling into self pity, perhaps saying things we don't mean and generally being the less intelligent, calm and centred people we otherwise are. At times like this we have been overtaken by our feelings and we lose control, regressing into animalistic, survival-based behaviour in the style of fight, flight and freeze.

Our survival instinct is designed to bypass our evolved thinking brain, to save our lives quickly in times of real danger. In ancient times this may have translated to running from wild animals. But in modern times it could be that we are enraged by drivers who cut us off in traffic, disrespectful neighbours, ineffective colleagues, badly behaved children and many other daily triggers. It could also be anxiety or anger triggered by our own thoughts and worries. At these times we are unable to focus on anything else. At best we overreact, saying things we wish we hadn't and later realising the error of our ways, hopefully in time to apologise. At worst, some may behave violently or self-sabotage. Terms like *emotional flooding* and *emotional hijack* have been used to describe this. At these times the parts of our brain responsible for logical, rational thinking are taken over by more primitive emotional- and survival-oriented brain regions.

THE AMYGDALA

In his book *Emotional Intelligence: Why it can matter more than IQ*, Daniel Goleman refers to this as 'the hijacking of the amygdala'. Goleman drew on the work of neuroscientist Joseph LeDoux and his discovery that the brain's signaling of strong emotions bypasses the rational neocortex to send a distress alert directly to the emotional amygdala, a small organ lying deep in the centre of our brain. When this happens, emotions grab our attention so that we are forced to react quickly because our thinking processes would quite simply be too slow.

At these times we lose control of our behaviour, with a tendency towards emotional outbursts, irrational behaviour and clumsy movement. Images of the perceived threat fill our minds; for example, we may 'see red' and visualise revenge, or urgently react to try to fix what we perceive needs fixing. Our minds can run film clips over and over again about all of this until the flooding subsides.

If the initial alert amounts to nothing, like if you startle at the sound of something and then realise that there is nothing there, the primitive brain quietens down and you are able to listen again to your 'high' brain. If you have been swept away in emotional flooding, however, it can take a while, around 30 minutes, to regain composure. We know that we have regained access to our 'high' brain when the appropriateness or inappropriateness of our reactions dawns on us and when we may realise the need to make amends.

If emotional flooding happens too regularly, the flood of stress hormones and self-sabotaging behaviour can be damaging to our bodies. It can also be damaging over time to our relationships if we make a habit of losing our cool, saying hurtful things and generally behaving badly. If you find yourself flooded often, look back in time for the original source of the feeling. It usually points to something unresolved. To help resolve this, refer to the emotions and body memory chapters in this book, which will guide you to a deeper enquiry into the history of emotional triggers.

⇒ YOUR BRAIN IN THE PALM OF YOUR HAND ⇐

Dr Daniel Siegel came up with a simple way of representing your brain in the palm of your hand. It is a handy reminder of your brain's integrative, optimal and mature functioning and offers a simple way to express the idea of *emotional hijack*. Make a fist with your thumb tucked inside the palm of your hand. Your wrist and palm represent your impulsive 'low' brain, your thumb curling inwards represents your emotional 'mid' brain and your fingers curling over your thumb represents your 'high' brain. The fingernails of these curled-over fingers that can touch into your palm represent your prefrontal cortex that faces the world and that produces integrative fibres to cohere the functioning of your brain as a whole.

This hand position represents a regulated brain that functions well. Now, keeping your thumb in place, open up your fingers. Dr Siegel refers to this as 'flipping your lid'. When you 'flip your lid' the rational, wise and regulatory part of your brain disengages from the emotional and impulsive parts of your brain. Emotions and impulses come to the fore and can override your ability to think clearly and respond mindfully. These are the times when you act rashly or lash out in ways you might regret later.

'Flipping your lid' The 'high' brain disengages from the 'mid' and 'low' brain with a tendency to act rashly and speak out emotionally.	Integrated, wise brain Fingers representing your rational, potentially wise and empathic 'high' brain are neatly containing your thumb, representing your emotional 'mid' brain and your wrist and palm representing your impulsive 'low' brain.

⇒ MINDFUL BODY MOMENT ⇐

A handy reminder of integrated, wise brain functioning

When you notice your emotions rising and you feel like you might be starting to 'flip your lid', hold the integrated brain hand model by closing your thumb into the palm of your hand and holding it there for a few moments or for as long as you need to. This can remind you to bring your rational, wise self forwards instead of 'flipping your lid'. Perhaps take a moment to get a feel for how this simple reminder can influence your mind, emotions and body in the moment.

Understanding this simple model gives you a basis for all stress management, whether acute or chronic. The intention is to develop your capacity for 'high' brain functioning. With acute stress, short, momentary interventions like holding this hand position can revive integrated brain functioning and a calmer, clearer outlook. When stress is chronic, momentary interventions like this one can provide some relief. To gain greater relief, it is important, perhaps with professional support, to address and resolve the reasons for chronic stress so that greater emotional resilience can be achieved. Life can also be a work in progress in which some degree of chronic stress might be part of our experience. It is still the case that we are better off when we have strategies, such as the ones offered in this book. They can help us manage daily stress by offering at least some relief and helping us to feel more in control.

⇒ MINDFUL BODY PROCESS ⇐

Recognising your style of losing control

The first step towards taking charge of your reactions is to be able to recognise and catch yourself in a moment of madness. This Mindful Body Process invites you to become familiar with your particular brand of 'flipping your lid' so that you can catch it when it occurs and more quickly 'close the lid' of your 'high' brain to guide yourself forwards.

We are creatures of habit with fairly predictable patterns of behaving. For example, do you shout and scream (the fight response)? Or do you storm away (the flight response)? Do you freeze or go blank (the freeze response)? Or perhaps you feel faint or sudden fatigue as if wanting to disappear, become invisible or deny that anything is going on. People draw on different strategies in different situations and with different people; you may sometimes freeze, and other times scream. Through observation we can come to recognise how consistent our response patterns can be.

The trigger

To get a clearer picture of your style of reacting, think of a time recently when you lost your cool. Take a moment to recall a specific moment as vividly as you can. What was the trigger? It might have been the end of a long day or demanding children; it might have been a really busy time at work and someone kept distracting you; it might have been feeling pushed too far by people around you. There can be any number of triggers, large and small.

The response

How did you feel? You might have felt irritated, upset, angry or anxious. Spend a few moments looking into your feelings. Does anything stand out? Where in your body do you experience these feelings most? What behaviours tend to go with these feelings? You may have pointed your finger or gesticulated madly; maybe you stood with arms folded or hands on your hips; or perhaps you stomped off or shouted loudly.

What happened?

What happened when you acted this way? How did the scenario unfold and how long did it last? How long did you take to recover and did you make amends afterwards? If so, what strategies did you or the other person use to resolve the situation, and how did that go? These situations flair up and then pass. Sometimes they resolve completely and other times they can remain simmering beneath the surface until the next trigger sets you off again. It is the flair-up that we are going to focus on a little more, now, to help you recognise it better in future. Recognising it and naming it can free you to move beyond it more quickly. In so doing you can regain access to your 'high' brain's perspective for some wise and compassionate input.

Name it

To find a name for your 'flipped out state', return to the memory of how you lost your cool. If you were to associate an image, perhaps an animal, to describe your reaction, what would it be? A roaring lion, a stomping elephant, a tortoise retreating into its shell? What comes to mind? Play with any image you like, to find one that feels like a good fit and then give it a name based on its characteristics.

Have fun with this exercise, as you recognise the animalistic instincts that can surface when your 'high' brain loses its control.

Then shift your perspective to remind yourself of your mature self. To help with this, recall a time you felt cool, calm, connected and collected. Allow the feeling of this memory to seep into your body and to shape your posture. Spend a few moments with this state to gain a clearer sense of it, noticing how you feel now and how your outlook might have changed. Perhaps also give this mature version of yourself a name, associating it with a descriptive word or image that can contrast with your previous less mature image of yourself.

For one final step, you are invited to juxtapose your mature and your 'flipped out' state. You can do so by taking on the characteristics of your 'flipped out' and mature states in alternation. Move from one to the other a few times to really notice the difference.

You might also be interested to consider what advice they might give to each other, considering that each might have value to add. Perhaps your 'flipped lid' self advises your calm self to be more confident and assertive, or more willing to ask for help, or to not try to do so much all at once. Perhaps your calm, collected self advises your 'flipped lid' self to be careful and hold back from doing harm, or to take a moment to consider how to use power wisely.

It is important to realise that your 'flipped lid' state serves a purpose. Perhaps this purpose is stepping into freedom for a few moments to counteract rigid self-control. Or it could give you a sense of power that you might not have access to otherwise, giving you the courage to effect change or set boundaries in a situation that you have struggled with.

The ultimate test of your ability to recognise your 'flipped lid' state will be in the days that follow this exploration when you hopefully are able to catch your reactions. With recognition you might say, 'Ah, hello, here you are again. What is really needed here? And how can I better use this energy?'

⇾ FINDING OUR WAY BACK FROM STRESS WITH BODY FIRST-AID ⇽

When overcome by stress, the sooner we can find our way back to calmer, clearer functioning, the better. To follow are some practical stress-relieving strategies to guide us back to aligning with our best self. The strategies are divided into three sections: The first section gives general body first-aid options to calm us and allow our minds to think more clearly. This can help with daily stress, whether you have a history chequered with lots of stress or whether you are generally happy and only experience stress now and again. Following this are specific recommendations for managing common causes of daily stress in a body-referenced way. The third section speaks to chronic stress and trauma. Following this are suggestions for Mind Body Moments that anyone can benefit from, no matter what your stress level is. These practices can support emotional resilience, mind-body integration and optimal brain functioning. For those who carry a backlog of stress, such as unresolved trauma, these practices are intended to complement, but not replace, professional intervention.

⇾ GENERAL BODY FIRST-AID STRATEGIES ⇽

Six-second rule

There is a window in which the rush of bio-chemicals triggered in the pre-emotional flooding time, such as adrenaline, begin to kick in. If not reacted to, this initial rush of urgent intensity and heightened focus will dissipate in three to six seconds. This is provided that you can hold off on reacting in that short time so that your reaction can quieten down enough to allow your thinking brain to kick in. Then you can be more considered in your response.

Intervening at the body level sends a message to your reptilian brain that you are safe and that you can relax. To follow are some ideas for taking charge in those first six seconds. Use whichever ones work best for you.

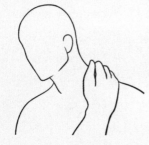

Take a few deep breaths when you catch yourself worked up

This is one way to prevent your amygdala from taking control and causing an emotional reaction. Step away for a few moments if need be, or ask for a few moments to regain your composure. Take your time to respond.

Use self-supporting touch

Massage a tense area of your body or hold your own hand to help you steady your emotional spike. The chapter about greeting your body with touch can offer you more ideas in this area.

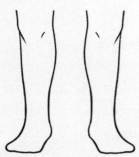

Centre and ground yourself

Stand evenly on your two feet or, if you are sitting, centre your weight over both hips. This encourages you to feel more balanced physically, which can translate into responding in a more balanced manner.

You can also stand or sit taller, as if reaching up out of your physical tensions and your emotions to observe yourself and your situation from a higher place. Doing so can help you to feel stronger in yourself, perhaps connecting you with your values and your ability to see the bigger picture. This can help you to respond more maturely.

Go for a walk or move your body in some way

Physical movement can interrupt emotional hijack escalation. It helps to keep your blood flowing and can give a physical outlet to the rush of feelings, allowing them to pass more quickly. If possible, you can suggest to the person who may have triggered these feelings, 'let's go for a walk and talk'.

BUY TIME

All of these strategies are essentially buying you time, even if just a few seconds, so that knee-jerk reactions can be sidelined in favour of more mature responses. You could also say something like, 'We are both triggered right now. Let's wait a few moments and then talk things through.' You could say the same to yourself when your mind is running wild and your emotions are boiling, such as, 'I am too triggered right now. I need to give myself time to think clearly.' Remember your survival reactions are much faster than your thinking processes, so you need a few moments, and the assurance of safety, to invite your rational and collaborative thinking to come back to the fore.

Clarify and label your emotions

While buying time it can be helpful to acknowledge your emotions. You might do so in your own mind, or out loud in the presence of others. For example, you might, say 'I feel angry', 'I am really upset', or even 'I feel so out of control'. Researcher Matthew Lieberman has shown that when people put words to their emotions the amygdala calms down almost instantly. It can give you a level of detachment that is necessary to allow your stress response to calm down so that your 'high' brain can add its intelligent perspective. Naming feelings can be relieving and can awaken compassion for yourself and perhaps for others, too, which can positively influence how you respond. Another name given to this practice is 'name it to tame it'. It has been found to work better for some people than for others. Give it a try. If it does not work for you, try another strategy.

Bring heart in and think again

Place your hand on your heart to feel connected with yourself and to convey sincerity. You can also, if you wish, imagine surrounding your feelings, and all the feelings in the room, with love. Then consider how to proceed. This can soften your eyes and your demeanor, which can send a signal of safety to the person you are with.

Watch your thoughts and ask 'Is it true?'

When caught up in emotional flooding it is likely that our outlook is negative, with a tendency to make assumptions and judgements about our situation. Especially with fear or anger, we can believe that something is true when it is not. One idea is to ask, 'Am I correct in thinking that . . . ?' Then be open to understanding things differently. If you are in an argument, sharing your thoughts and fears might be the only way to check assumptions. Once you have listened to each other's truth, you probably will be in a better position to consider how you can resolve your situation and perhaps support each other in the process too.

IF YOU GET STUCK

The power of distraction

Do something completely different. Go for a walk, work on something else for a while, try another angle, choose another activity. Try anything in order to break the emotional flood and bring in new perspectives and energy. Then return with this new perspective to share insights and make amends if need be.

Exercise when you get a chance

Going to the gym or exercising in your own way can release pent-up stress, opening you to calmer, clearer thinking and insights. In the moment 'walking and talking' can help keep your blood flowing and your stress hormones at bay, to some extent. Exercise allows you to release accumulated stress, and can reconnect you with feeling strong in your body and mind. You may also gain new insights and perspective. Do share your new thoughts with others you may be in conflict with, as you seek to resolve and learn from the incident and buffer against similar triggers in future.

Find something funny about your behaviour or situation

You might ask, 'I wonder if we will laugh about this one day?' There is nothing like humour to diffuse tension. The trick is bringing it in appropriately, at the right time (not too soon) and not at anybody's expense.

POST-EMOTIONAL HIJACK

If you have been swept away in the throes of an amygdala hijack, with your mind and body thoroughly flooded by stress hormones, it can take some time, like around 30 minutes, for your nervous system to calm down. A sign of emotional flooding might be when you feel so upset or angry that your situation feels like it is spiraling out of control. At these times it is wise to wait before trying to problem-solve or pick up a conversation again. Your ability to listen, negotiate, discuss, be empathic, and engage constructively, depends on you regaining your composure. Similarly, the people you might be with also might need time to recover, too. So, if you find yourself in an impasse, asking to speak in half an hour, for example, is for the benefit of the other person as well as yourself and can lead to the best outcome. It is helpful to agree on when and where you will speak or at least check in again. It can be reassuring to know that the situation will be addressed. Then it is important to follow up with this and reconnect at some point in order to prevent prolonged emotional flooding.

With practice and with the skill of mindfulness you can recover more quickly from these moments and generally become less prone to being emotionally overthrown.

TARGETING SPECIFIC STRESS

Time stress and holding time in the body

Life can be relentless and demanding. If you are a stay-at-home parent or a working parent, an employee, a business owner or a student, or even a child, the demands of modern, fast-paced living can take their toll on your resilience and health. Our relationship to time is something we can play with to cope better with the many things we juggle in our lives.

It can be helpful to reflect on how you hold the sense of time in your body. You might consider, 'Do I often feel tense and rushed?' 'Is this a repeated feeling for me, such as leaving things to the last minute?' Some people have a habit of responding to life in a rush, even when it might not be necessary. You might also consider if your level of physical tension, and your state of mind, help or hinder your ability to be calm and timeous? When our 'lids are flipped' even slightly, we can add unnecessary stress, strain and insensitive communication to our lives. Sometimes all it takes is catching ourselves in a worked-up, chaotic state, and intervening to allow calmer, clearer functioning to return.

Once aware of our general relationship with time, it can awaken our curiosity to explore new ways of being in relation to time. We might pause to reflect, plan and prioritise before acting. We might pause now and again to ease physical tension with body first-aid strategies so that we are in a better state of mind and body to carry out all that we need to. These kinds of strategies can make our lives easier, helping us to complete what we need to, more calmly and timeously.

When feeling under time pressure, it can also be helpful to ask, 'What's the worst that can happen?' For some this can ease personal pressure and bring a breath of fresh air as you realise that the worst scenario is perhaps not as catastrophic as you might have believed. To turn this into a Mindful Body Moment, you could take 30 seconds or so to invite the feeling of relief to seep into your body and brain for a lasting effect, before you return to the task at hand.

Anticipatory stress

There are different kinds of anticipatory stress. It can be experienced in the short term as a natural part of learning and personal growth. You might experience this when you embark on a new life path, such as starting a new job, opening your own business, being newly divorced or starting on a course of study. This short-term anticipatory stress can be motivating or terrifying, depending on the moment. The second kind of anticipatory stress is a more frequent or chronic tendency to worry about every little thing.

Both live in our imagination and are receptive to change through visualisation processes. They are both helped by learning to live more in the present, as opposed to in our thoughts, feelings and beliefs about what *might* happen.

Try the following imagination strategies to find out what works best for you. To ground your imagination in your body and brain it is recommended that you hold the helpful outcome in your posture for a few moments, perhaps adding some supportive touch. This can clear your mind and free you to get on with planning, preparing and acting on what you need to without as much emotional interference.

Case study 1: Imagine a good outcome

Opening a new restaurant was always Luke's dream and was something very close to his heart. When he finally did achieve this, he was swamped by anticipatory stress and anxiety about people criticising his food and not liking the look of the restaurant. Luke was encouraged to visualise kind, appreciative eyes receiving him. As he played with this image, he let the feelings sink into his body and affect his mind. His body felt warmer as he did so and he felt he could breathe more easily. On being asked to find a particular part of his body that noticeably related to this experience, he chose his eyes. He described the feeling of his eyes softening as if sinking back into their sockets all the way down, to connect with his heart. He used this reminder, from eyes to heart, for a few moments whenever he thought people were rejecting his restaurant. This kind of practice can challenge old beliefs that people will automatically be judgemental and hostile.

Case study 2: Imagine the worst-case scenario

Cindy was really stressed about an exam. She decided to tackle her stress with humour and asked herself, 'What's the worst that could happen?' When she thought through what might happen, she was surprised to realise how unlikely it was that the exam would go so badly. And even if it did, she could take the exam again or perhaps, in the worst-case scenario, give up on following her career path and choose another one that, in the long run, might work out better for her. On allowing the feelings of relief to sink into her mind and body, she felt more ready to get on with studying for the exam, with her worries left behind, and a giggle when her worst-case scenarios popped back in mind. Fleshing out a worst-case scenario in your mind does not necessarily add to your stress, instead it can ease it. You might realise, 'OK, I can deal with that.' Or, 'Is that really so bad?' This realisation can help you breathe easier and focus more clearly.

Using your senses to tune in to the present moment

Another way to support the tendency to worry is to take breaks in your day, to reset your senses to focus on the present moment. To do so you could take a Mindful Body Moment of just a minute or two, to take in your surroundings afresh. Spend a few moments noticing through each of your five senses. Notice what you see, what you hear, what you smell, what your skin feels, such as the temperature of the air, and what taste is in your mouth. This can help to orient your attention to the now, and open you to a new sense of being alive in the moment.

Or, to enhance your sensory experience, you could go for a walk during a break and experience your surroundings through your five senses, in the fresh air. If you are prone to chronic worry, spending as much time out in nature as you can, perhaps choosing outdoor hobbies and sports, can go a long way to reminding you of the beauty and wonder of the world. This can shift your attention away from your worries and promote inner peace and calm.

Emotional and physical stress

Stress can also be triggered by unresolved emotional baggage and by physical demands, ailments and injuries. For support with these kinds of stress, refer to later chapters dedicated to working with emotions or ailments and injuries respectively.

Arguments

When we are faced with someone in the throes of emotional flooding it is easy to also get swept away in the flood. Daniel Goleman refers to this as complementary emotional hijacking. It is a key relationship skill to be able to notice when others are emotionally flooded and to manage not to be swept up in their emotional state. Then at least one of you is able to see reason and stay centred and grounded. If both of you are emotionally flooded there is no logical intelligence left in the room. When in the throes of complementary emotional flooding, the other person can feel like your enemy and nothing can be resolved until one of you (or both of you) finds your way back to a calmer, clearer state. Albert Einstein's quote rings true here that 'you can't solve a problem from the state of mind in which it exists'.

Realising that others also succumb to emotional flooding is a good starting point. Then, using body first-aid strategies suggested earlier can buy you enough time to keep your own cool and to encourage the person in front of you to calm down too. To follow is another helpful strategy that can help.

Sincere listening and 'feeling felt'

Many of us live in a chronic state of stress, perhaps overwhelmed and braced against the world because of past challenges. Irritation, anger, resistance and anxiety are some common side effects. To a greater or lesser extent this means that many of us live in some degree of emotional flooding, which makes us more reactive to life's annoyances. When you talk to someone who is caught up in even a small emotional flood it is no different to talking to a cornered animal. If your style of trying to get through to them is even vaguely confrontational you will simply invite resistance or defensive behaviour. In his book *Just Listen: Discover the Secret to Getting Through to Absolutely Anyone* psychiatrist Mark Goulston explains what our brains need in order to move from emotional flooding and resistance to being able to listen again. What is needed is heartfelt, authentic and agenda-less listening.

From his work with suicidal and violent individuals, and as a provider of training in hostage negotiation for the police and FBI, Goulston speaks of success hinging entirely on guiding the person up from the reptile to the mammal to what he calls the 'primate' (equivalent to neo-mammalian) brain. His techniques involve listening, asking for more information, mirroring and reflecting back what the person has said. When you do so, the other person not only feels listened to, they also feel understood, seen and felt. As a result they are more likely to open up to you. You might need to put aside your own feelings and start this process when in an argument. The outcome can be a pleasant surprise if the other person softens and starts to listen to your perspective in order to work things through.

Goulston refers to 'feeling felt' as a necessary ingredient to add to your listening. Having others 'feel felt' is a function of mirror neurons that Goulston believes are an important aspect of moving people up to their more evolved brains. Mirror neurons are what make you squirm when watching your favourite soccer team miss a goal or when you see someone hurt themself. Mirror neurons have also been called empathy neurons because they allow you to feel into someone else's experience as if it were your own.

In the case of conflict resolution, utilising mirror neurons allows you to feel into the reality of the person in front of you, as if you are standing in their shoes. To achieve this, try adopting something of their posture, gestures, movement quality and emotional tone. All of this can help you feel into their reality more clearly and reflect empathy in a kinesthetic way. This shows them that you not only see them, but that you also feel their experience. When done sensitively this can convey that you really are present with the other person, that you see them and get them, or that you are genuinely seeking to understand where they are coming from. Squarely facing the person and maintaining eye contact can also convey that you are giving them your full attention, which can be reassuring. But be careful that you don't mirror their emotional state (such as anxiety or rage) to such an extent that you can't tell yourself from them. By being so emotional yourself, you may exacerbate the other person's emotional overwhelm or panic. To help you avoid this, you might explore speaking slowly and clearly for a calming effect. This may also encourage you to be mindful in your choice of words.

This kind of empathic mirroring of another person's reality, together with heartfelt listening can, according to Goulston, create an irresistible biological urge that pulls the person towards you, allowing them to be open to your ideas, melting away the state of emotional flooding. This, in turn, evolves the brain regions so that the person you are with can respond to you with reason, sensibility and perhaps even with heart.

⇒ NOTES ABOUT CHRONIC STRESS AND TRAUMA ⇐

Dr Daniel Siegel's 'Window of Tolerance' is a helpful term when considering the topic of chronic stress and trauma. It refers to the optimal state for brain and physiological functioning while awake. You can think of it as a zone in which you feel able to meet the demands of life in a relatively calm, collected and connected way. If you become emotional, you are able to soothe and regulate your experience. You are also able to be empathic and supportive of others. In this zone your brain can effectively receive, process and integrate information. You are able to think rationally and creatively, reflect on experience and make decisions relatively calmly without feeling overwhelmed or withdrawn. It is a state of healthy emotional resilience.

When stress or threat levels rise higher than you can tolerate, or when you feel like you are losing control, survival responses of fight, flight, freeze or faint force you out of your 'window'. Dr Siegel describes this as moving into either rigidity or chaos. Before attempting to talk things through or make sense of a situation, it is important to find your way back into your 'window', otherwise stress and conflict can simply spiral out of control. Your body can help you track and manage your experience to help you back into your 'window'. With chronic stress or trauma, professional support can be key to releasing and integrating really distressing experiences, so that you are able to return to healthy levels of emotional resilience.

Depending on your life experience, natural temperament, and experience with mindfulness, each person will have a different 'window of tolerance'. Some have a narrow 'window' causing them to experience emotions and life intensely, and in a way that is often hard to manage. For these people life can feel like an emotional rollercoaster ride. Other people have a wider 'window' giving them the ability to handle greater emotional intensity and function well under stress and pressure. Mindfulness is one way to naturally widen our 'window of tolerance'.

The key to remaining in or returning to our 'window of tolerance', is feeling safe and supported. The more safe and supported we feel, the more we can grow our emotional resilience and resolve any backlog of stress that we may have accumulated. Most of us move into and out of our 'windows' as a part of life's journey of ups and downs. As we become more emotionally resilient our 'window' widens so that we can feel more present with life, and more stable. This allows us to live within our 'window' more often and when we are triggered we are able to return to it relatively quickly.

ABOUT TRAUMA

Trauma can take two basic forms. One is an event or series of events that shatters our ability to cope. The other kind of trauma is developmental, where our basic emotional needs were not sufficiently met when we were babies or children, to the extent that the absence of this support seriously impacts our ability to feel safe in life. Either way, trauma and the extreme stress that it causes throw the nervous system out of balance to such an extent that a person is easily triggered into survival mode by any small stressor. The world feels like an unsafe place as their 'window of tolerance' shrinks to become very narrow or inflexible. This means that they may see and react to real or imagined threats many times, even in a single day, by fighting, fleeing, freezing or becoming lethargic (as an expression of a faint response). Mental health issues like depression and anxiety are common as are symptoms of post-traumatic stress like flashbacks, nightmares, dissociation and memory issues.

Finding a 'window of tolerance' under these conditions usually requires psychological support. This can provide a safe space for people to begin to engage with, and process, very painful, challenging feelings. In so doing, a healing journey can be facilitated towards slowly expanding our 'window of tolerance'.

To complement professional support for chronic stress or trauma, follow the Mindful Body Moments below, which can be incorporated into daily life. They are intended to be playful, active ways to encourage mind-body integration, promote vitality and support emotional resilience.

⇒ TWO MINDFUL BODY MOMENTS FOR ALL ⇐

Improving stress management through body awareness

SCANNING FOR TENSION

Making a habit of freeing your body of tension by checking in with it from time to time through your day can go a long way to help you manage and reduce stress build-up. To do so you might notice where you habitually hold stress in your body. You probably know the areas that speak to you most in tension or aches. Then you could pause now and again to breathe into tight or tired areas, stretching and, if you wish, briefly massaging or holding the areas supportively, to loosen and energise yourself.

You could also scan your body from head to toe to fill any gaps in your awareness as you notice and inhabit your body more fully. Moving from head to toe, you could breathe into each part of your body in turn and perhaps use some movement, stretching and self-supporting touch as you go, for an energising, refreshing effect on your body and mind. If you notice areas of tension you will probably adjust your posture and take deeper breaths to feel freer. It could also be that each part of your body is infused with energy of its own, such that when more of your body is included in your awareness it can enhance your overall sense of vitality.

INCLUDING MORE OF YOUR BODY IN AWARENESS

What does it mean to include more of your body in your everyday awareness? For example, in your habitual style of walking you might predominantly use your legs and your arms in a particular way and hold your head at a particular angle. Next time you walk, it could be interesting to play with this. You could experiment with walking just with your legs (as can happen when caught up in your thoughts), with very little upper body movement. How does this feel? Then experiment with including more of your body. You might move your arms with your stride or allow your whole body to become more involved with your movement somehow, as if you were a dancer moving with synchronised flow. How does it feel to move with fuller body integration and awareness? Also, while exercising, such as running, you could explore including different parts of your body in your awareness, to notice how this might contribute to your physical ease, mobility, energy, performance and state of mind.

You could also play with styles of walking that you might enjoy. You could try walking like your favourite film character or walking in a graceful or dignified manner. You could explore walking with strength or rhythmically, determinedly or gently or with any quality you like. What walking style do you like best today? Or how about trying to walk in a way that prints peace and serenity on the earth – a practice endorsed by the Vietnamese monk and peace activist, Thich Nhat Hanh. Play with it.

By bringing more body awareness into your natural movement, you bring more of yourself into your moment. In extending this practice you could also consider bringing more of yourself into your life and what this might offer you? What parts of yourself might you be afraid to include and for what reasons? Is there a way that you could include some new part of yourself, even in some small way, into your walking and your life? In the words of Susan Aposhyan, in her book *Natural Intelligence*, 'including more of us always shifts our perspective and our creative resources. If you feel stuck in your life, try checking in with your body. Notice what you are ignoring and consciously invite it. New solutions inevitably arise.'

CHAPTER 5

Emotions and Turning to the Body

All emotions are reflected in the body and mind.
Envy and fear cause the face to pale. Love makes it glow.

PARAMAHANSA YOGANANDA

The key to emotional wellbeing, emotional healing and emotional resilience is listening to your emotions, noticing how they stir your body, mind and spirit, and engaging with them instead of resisting or denying them. 'It's as simple as noticing how you feel and then having a conversation with your feelings, in which *you* do most of the listening,' says Ann Weiser Cornell, author of *The Power of Focusing*.

By turning to your body you can notice how emotions are experienced through sensations, body posture and distinct characteristics. Your body language is the raw data of your emotions expressed through physical sensations, like heaviness or jitters in your belly or tightness in your jaw or a sinking feeling in the pit of your stomach. This gives you tangible material to engage with. Spending time being curious and caring about your emotions, especially in such a visceral way, can make a world of difference. Not only can it help you to acknowledge your feelings more objectively, you can also begin to appreciate that they are there for a reason. You are then also in a good position to be able to respond supportively to how you feel in service of emotional healing and resilience. This kind of attitude towards your emotions can also translate to being able to give the same respectful presence to the emotions of others.

This chapter begins with the skill of characterising emotions for assistance in working with them. It moves on to explore emotions as energy that can be experienced in the body. To end is a guided Mindful Body Process for when you might wish to work through a specific emotion, in-depth, towards emotional insight and transformation.

⇒ EMOTIONAL DRAMAS, EMOTIONAL CHARACTERS ⇐

Emotions can play out as epic dramas in our lives. This gives us a theatrical way of working with our emotions, as if they are characters acting in a drama. By visualising this you can notice how you are feeling, how your feelings shape your body and mind and how they play into the dramas of your life. This can be applied in many ways such as in decision-making or to turn your experience around when you feel irritated, upset or jealous. The tools of this section can guide you to resolve and evolve emotional challenges and build a stronger, more trusting relationship with your emotional world.

MANY EMOTIONS, MANY CHARACTERS

Some names used by different authors to describe this kind of emotional characterisation are 'sub-personalities', 'voices' or 'parts'. For example, Sigmund Freud introduced an id, ego and superego. Carl Jung brought us the idea of archetypes that he believed reside in the collective unconscious of all people. In Carol Pearson's book *The Hero Within*, she expands on Jung's ideas, referring to specific archetypes of the innocent, orphan, warrior, caregiver, seeker, lover, destroyer, creator, ruler, magician, sage and fool. Each of these archetypes has a developmental task to complete in their evolutionary journey.

Dr Eric Berne's Transactional Analysis identifies three ego states that adults can move between. These include a parent, a child and an adult state. Dr Stephen Karpman's Drama Triangle offers us the victim, the rescuer and the persecutor that exist in relation to each other, especially in conflict. Alcoholics Anonymous uses The Dysfunctional Family System, with roles assumed in dysfunctional family systems where addictive behaviour is present. These roles include addict, enabler, scapegoat or the one who acts out, jester, lost or invisible child who could also be a good child, family hero or the responsible one, and the placater or caretaker role.

You can get creative and come up with your own fitting names for different characters that you might play in life. With attention, you can notice how each character has its own distinct emotional tone, behavioural tendencies, way of thinking and outlook.

Whatever they are called, they characterise you in ways that can be predictable. Once you get to know the cast of your usual characters, who make appearances in your life, you can find out what triggers each of them, what different 'characters' need and how to use each to your benefit. You can discover which 'characters' like to take the lead in your life and which can be brought forward to offer you a more balanced experience. Or you can simply pause and enjoy the quality of your feelings and the 'character' with you in a particular moment.

EMOTIONAL BIOCHEMISTRY

Just like the personality types of the previous chapter, emotions also create their own distinct bio-chemistry, which changes according to how you feel. This is because, from a neuroscientific perspective, emotions are bio-chemical reactions throughout the body and brain that trigger the release of molecules that create the feelings of emotions. These in turn affect your body language and your outlook.

According to the neuroscientist Dr Candace Pert, emotions are quantum-level triggers for changes from one sub-personality or state of being to the next. She believes that understanding all of our multiple emotional states as if they are sub-personalities can help us to understand many troublesome problems, including drug addiction and weight control, or anything that challenges us and that involves making decisions. The question is which sub-personality is making decisions for you at this time? For example, is it your angel or your devil? Once you can find compassion, acceptance, perhaps forgiveness and integration of all your emotional experiences, then a new state can emerge of 'selves-esteem', as Dr Pert describes it. So you grow your overall sense of self-worth knowing that each part of you has an important role to play.

WE ARE ALL MULTI-DIMENSIONAL

Your various emotional 'characters' playing out in your daily life make you a multi-dimensional person, positive at times, even-keel at times and down at times. You might be a loving, nurturing person at times, or a chatty, sociable person; a productive, efficient person; a grumpy, miserable, overloaded person, or a frustrated, irritable person, all depending on what is going on for you at the time, and how you are feeling.

In an earlier chapter you met the 'flipped lid' version of yourself. In another chapter you might have discovered personality-related aspects of yourself such as being bold, nurturing, thoughtful or excitable. On reflection you could probably identify more versions of yourself that you could give fitting names to, such as an inner teacher; a carefree inner child; a mature, wise self; an invisible or hidden you, a winner, a loser, a victim, a warrior, an inner critic, etc. Each has its own characteristic feeling tone, posture and state of mind. Some feeling tones have a history dating back many years and some might have evolved more recently. Some emotional tendencies can be inherited and might date back through many generations. Together, all of your emotional expressions form part of the big picture of who, and how, you are in life.

Reflection

How many versions of you have shown up recently? To help you, think of the various emotional ups and downs that you have moved through lately and how you have behaved.

Which version of yourself has played a leading role lately and how has that been working for you?

What kind of character might be helpful to you now, and why?

⟫ THREE MINDFUL BODY PROCESSES ⟪

For emotional support and resilience

To follow are a few practical applications of emotional characterisation told through true stories. The intended outcome is always emotional insight and emotional resilience. Included are processes to assist with decision-making, dealing with emotions by consulting a 'higher self' for guidance, and working through our reactions to others to gain personal insight.

For those wishing for support with depression and anxiety, note that they will receive attention in the chapter called 'Healing old patterns, enhancing vitality'. Look out for the Mindful Body Reflection in that chapter that focuses on depression and anxiety.

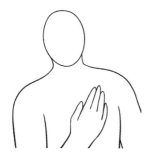

A HEAD-HEART DIALOGUE TO ASSIST WITH DECISION-MAKING

The classic head-heart battle can be a source of great stress in decision-making. Or it can be used consciously to your advantage if you allow each to be heard and contribute to the decision-making process. This dialogue between head and heart can be insightful because you have the opportunity to weigh up the pros and cons of each and find your way to integrate the perspectives of both. Here is an example of how a head-heart dialogue played out in Sally's decision-making, and her process of following through on the decision that she made.

Case study 3: Head and heart

Sally had a big life decision to make about whether or not to move back to her home country after many years of being away. During our psychotherapy work together, many of our conversations centred around two perspectives: The one perspective was a rational 'head' perspective used for addressing logical matters during her decision-making process, and later for planning in a practical and organised way for her relocation; the second perspective was an emotional 'heart' perspective. This represented all of her feelings about making the difficult decision to leave what felt like home at the time. Her heart had known for a long time that she wanted to move back to her previous home to be closer to her parents, especially as she was considering having her first child. Her heart feelings were strong about this and she felt torn because she would be moving away from the rich and rewarding life that she had built for herself in the country that had been her home for the last few years. Ultimately her heart won out and she set a date to move home. Her heart continued to occupy a seat in our therapy room as a space for exploring her emotional needs and speaking about her emotional experience. This sometimes felt overwhelming for her, particularly when she started moving towards her departure date. An example of her 'heart needs' included making quality time for all of her friends and acquaintances, to say her goodbyes. She also decided to visit her favourite places each weekend leading up to her departure, as her way of saying goodbye to the city that she had come to love. There was also heartfelt acknowledgement of how she had matured personally and professionally over the last years. 'Head' and 'heart' themes appeared so often that two seats were regularly set up in the therapy room to accommodate them. This also provided Sally with the opportunity to step out of the emotional intensity of the process when it all felt like too much. To accommodate this, we allocated a neutral seat for Sally to sit in at the start and at the end of our sessions and any time she felt she needed it. This seat acted as a place where Sally could look in on what was unfolding in her world, as an observer. This also made space for noticing other aspects of her life that might otherwise have been ignored in the consuming head-heart process of her major life transition.

In Sally's 'head-heart' process of decision-making, each perspective offered important contributions that led to an integration of logic and reason with heart and emotion. The outcome was that she felt peaceful about her decision, satisfied that she had honoured her feelings every step of the way and that she had been well organised in wrapping up her life in one country and preparing for her new life in another country. She kept up a daily to-do list for months before leaving and made space for her feelings along the way. These feelings included loss and excitement, fear and love, resolve and feeling overwhelmed. It was a rich and busy time. Then the time of her departure came, and, with loving tears, she closed a special chapter in her life, with clarity, knowing why she had chosen to take this next step.

EMOTIONS AND CONSULTING A 'HIGHER SELF' FOR GUIDANCE

In her book *Everything You Need to Know to Feel Go(o)d*, Dr Candace Pert shares her belief that the key to successful therapy is training yourself to come from a highest possible 'observer' or witness perspective. This can be seen as your 'higher self' that can be likened to accessing your 'high' brain, as referred to in the earlier chapter on stress. It is a version of yourself that aligns with noble virtues and that only wants the best for you.

A higher perspective can expand our awareness and can open us to mature, clear thinking not always available in our usual state of consciousness. This can offer us benefits such as greater self-acceptance, perspective, hope, vision, comfort and insight, in relation to our life experience. To add to the material offered in the chapter on stress, here is another opportunity for reflection on this 'higher self' as well as an example of how one woman applied this life skill in her work environment.

Reflection

Take a moment to consider what your higher self feels and looks like. It might be you in some higher, more compassionate form or you as an older, wiser version of yourself. Or it might be a figure that you can call to mind when you wish to consult higher wisdom, such as a loving, supportive person in your life, now or from your past. Or perhaps it is a spiritual or angelic presence or a fantasy creature that represents ultimate wisdom, for you to consult in times of need. Spend a few moments developing the image of your higher self as clearly as you can.

How do you feel when your higher self is around? Notice how your body responds. How is your breathing and your posture affected, and how does this influence your state of mind as well as how you feel? Perhaps ask your higher self to give you some advice about a current challenge. Then listen and wait for a response that might appear as words or an image or a feeling. Or a new idea might spring to mind. Be open to what comes. If you are not sure about what you have received, perhaps walk into your day open to how you might view your experiences differently when you carry this higher perspective with you. You might do so through your posture or by holding a word in mind that feels inspiring, such as dignity, trust or love.

In one woman's example, she created a 'wise' role to help her relax and be more effective at work. Using chairs to help distinguish each version of herself at first, she learned to step out of a physically tense and mentally harsh inner-critic 'seat' that she had learned from her critical mother. She also practised stepping out of a 'seat' or a role characterised by low self-esteem and a slouching, heavy-feeling posture. By contacting earlier life memories of feeling this way, she discovered that these feelings stemmed back to feeling vulnerable and never good enough as an overweight young girl. She found it comforting to realise that she could step out of the roles represented by the chairs. She also found comfort in the knowledge that she could return to them if she wished to at a later time, to explore and seek to resolve these old and distressing feelings, perhaps in therapy. Instead of all these feelings vying for her attention as she made her way through her day, she discovered her ability to separate them and step into and out of them at will.

She found great relief in stepping into her 'wise self' as she prepared for business meetings as well as for conversations with her mother. This helped her to think more clearly and constructively and to be more relaxed and upright, as opposed to feeling consumed by self-deprecating feelings and frustrations. This woman had been referred by her manager for work-related counseling because of feedback that her high levels of anxiety were interfering with her ability to be effective at work. In particular, this anxiety was interfering with her ability to communicate clearly with her colleagues. Feedback from colleagues, in the weeks that followed our sessions, was that they noticed a marked improvement in her ability to contain her anxiety in meetings, and that she appeared to generally be working more efficiently.

LIFE LESSONS LEARNED THROUGH OUR REACTIONS TO OTHERS

People who trigger and annoy you only get to you because they can represent a quality in you that is not well developed. For some people it might be vulnerability and for others it might be assertiveness or confidence. You may have spent years sweeping particular feelings under the carpet perhaps because it was not received well in your family or in your community or social circle. The same goes for people you place on a pedestal and those you envy. They can represent qualities about yourself that are either not fully formed or that are aspirational. In the case of envy, the longer you project these qualities onto others (perhaps their success, their ability to be affectionate, their comfort in their own skin or other), the more you keep yourself in a lower position and at those times, not able to live fully in your own life.

It is a common experience to value certain parts of our personalities and devalue or dislike others. Fritz Perls, who was the pioneer of Gestalt Psychology, refers to people having 'holes' in their psyche. These holes appear when we deny and project parts of ourselves onto others. Our holes can become our pitfalls. Claiming back these split- or disowned parts and filling them, gives us the opportunity to feel whole and more fulfilled. Debbie Ford, in her book *The Dark Side of the Light Chasers* suggests that our world is holographic and that everyone and everything is a mirror. We are always seeing reflections of ourselves in others. So, if we choose to, we can look at who emotionally affects us as an invitation to uncover a hidden or judged aspect of ourselves. This can be a catalyst for personal growth and can lead us to claim back useful traits and gain greater self-acceptance.

Case study 4: An irritation turned aspiration

At the start of our work together, Janet admitted to feeling unfulfilled in her life, at times to the point of despair. At the time Janet was a successful businesswoman, wife and mother of two teenage children. She carried a chronic knot in her chest. On exploring this as a 'character', it became a man, standing tall with hands on hips as if standing guard. What was he guarding? She did not know. She just knew that he was tough and that he despised 'crybabies'. She could not remember when she last cried. 'Just get on with it' was her motto. This 'character' reminded her of her father, whom she strived to please.

During our conversations she informed me that her sister-in-law was coming to visit. She despised her sister-in-law, which was apparent by her rolling her eyes and flicking her hand in disdain. 'This is all I need now!' This raised my curiosity about what disowned qualities her sister-in-law might represent in her and whether this might show us what lived behind the tough 'guarding' of the character with the knot in her chest. I asked her to describe her sister-in-law. She described her as irritating, irresponsible and laidback. On being encouraged to adopt her sister-in-law's posture and mannerisms, she slouched back in her seat. At first this felt uneasy and she laughed at how strange this felt for her. I asked her what it could give her life if she could be a bit more laidback. Some of her responses included: 'She takes no responsibility. She has it easy!' and 'I would love it if I could take it easier now and again.' 'Everyone around her takes care of her. I wish I could be taken care of a bit, too.' 'She lives in an escapist world.' On reflection, this all encapsulated a sense of freedom for her that she longed for. Her mother came to mind during this conversation. Her mother also lived a carefree, seemingly irresponsible life, similar to her sister-in-law's in some ways, although with the addition of some flamboyance. Janet longed for her life to feel exciting and free. 'But she left us...' Her mother had walked out on her family when she was young, except for occasional visits, leaving her father as a single parent.

At this point tears began to flow. A whole new vulnerability appeared as she hunched forwards over her arms with her head down. Later we allocated a seat to this new 'character', which represented her younger self. Around the time that her mother walked out she was a scared little girl. Her father had not been able to offer emotional support, probably because he too was struggling emotionally. As a result, Janet learned to hide her sadness away, and then eventually to lock it away forever so she could be tough for her father. It became obvious that this was the origin of why she could not stand adult 'crybabies'. 'Just get over it and get on with it.' But she had never truly got over it.

As our conversations continued, I wanted to get to know the little girl better. It came out that this little girl loved dressing up in clothes from a big chest that belonged to her mother. 'I still love clothes,' she shared. The next consideration was how to make this useful to her life now. She had considered being an image consultant some years before, although she did not know how to go about it or how to make it financially viable, especially as she was the breadwinner in her family and only had experience working in her current industry. We spoke about the possibility of including her love of fashion into her life in some small way. We considered a few options for taking this love of clothes to a new level. For a start, she liked the idea of buying some items of clothing on her overseas work travels for selling locally and informally. This would allow her to test out business ideas while still keeping up her current work.

By using Janet's response to her sister-in-law, and then her idealised mother, she could guide herself back to a sense of being carefree and doing what she loved – her love of clothes. Both offered clues for how she might feel more fulfilled in her life. As our meetings continued, Janet developed a vision and set goals for herself to include some of what she loved in her life. She felt excited for the first time in a long time about something related to work. It gave her something to look forward to while she continued working in her current job.

A couple of months later, Janet's husband was offered permanent employment. He had not had stable work for many years, leading to Janet's family depending on her salary. This meant that the pressure was lifted from Janet. As a result Janet was able to reduce her work hours to allow her more time to invest in her new ideas. Even though there were still good days and challenging days, her energy and spirits were lifted and her confidence in her new ideas grew. This motivated her to continue along her new path of reclaiming a long-lost part of her true nature and making space to integrate it in her life.

FOR YOUR REFLECTION

Who triggers you? What is it about that person that you don't like? Do these qualities remind you of someone or a time in your life?

Might these be qualities that you do not allow in yourself? If your irritation could be showing you an area for personal growth, what could it be?

Can you find forgiveness or patience for the shortcomings of yourself and others? Breathe, feel into and perhaps use some movement to express what is evoked in you when you consider this? How could this add value in your life even in some small way?

WHO DO YOU PLACE ON A PEDESTAL? WHO DO YOU IDEALISE?

Idealisation, or being in awe of others, also represents an aspect of yourself, perhaps an underdeveloped aspect, that you have projected onto someone else. If you can identify what you admire in others then you can consider how to develop these qualities in yourself. In Debbie Ford's words: 'Instead of fixating on someone else's brilliance, find ways to develop and demonstrate your own.'

Reflection

Think of someone in your life, or perhaps a person in your community or in the media, who you really admire. What is it about them that intrigues you? What qualities do they have that you might want to develop in yourself? Is it confidence, genuine kindness, caring, the ability to show vulnerability with dignity, admirable leadership skills, calmness under pressure? Choose what feels most fitting and breathe these qualities into your body. If you were to step into these aspirational qualities and own them, how might they help you in your life at this time? Remember that you only admire someone who is a mirror for something underdeveloped inside of you, or that you have undermined.

⇒ THE ENERGY OF EMOTIONS ⇐

Emotions are essentially how you are touched and moved by life. You might feel noticeably emotional at times or you might move through your day with an undercurrent of feelings. These emotions or the undercurrent of feelings alter your body language, your outlook and your behaviour. Emotions also bring energy with them, energy for you to be present with and to embody, and energy that is ever ebbing and flowing, never standing still and never lasting forever in one emotional state. Instead of resisting, reacting or withdrawing, you can try to remain present to the experience of your feelings. This means that you allow the energy of different emotions to touch and move you as you breathe with them, feel them, and value them as feedback about your experience. Perhaps you are aware of what needs attention in yourself, your relationships, or in your world. The energy of emotions can also motivate and energise you to do what you need to – perhaps adjusting your attitude or saying or doing something that feels important, or perhaps finding a creative outlet for your feelings. To follow are some basic emotional states and the energy that they bring. But before exploring the energies of different emotions, let's pause to introduce the endpoints of your body. This can encourage the outward flow of emotions so that you can feel perhaps safer and more confident in exploring your emotions.

⇛ MINDFUL BODY MOMENT ⇚

Awareness of body endpoints to assist the flow and release of emotional energy

This Mindful Body Moment can increase your sense of inner strength and ability to support yourself from the inside out. It does so by engaging end points of your body that assist with the discharge of your nervous system and emotional energy. Doing so can help you stand taller and stronger while emotionally charged, such as when you feel angry or afraid. It can also allow emotions to flow through you more freely for times when, for example, you might be feeling sad.

We all have probably experienced spontaneous moments when our bodies shudder, shake, twitch or jolt as a quick burst of energy moves through us. Energy can also pass through us in waves. These are signs that your nervous system is discharging energy. This energy could come from your emotions, stress build-up, or follow a state of shock. Energy can also discharge at seemingly random times as our minds and bodies navigate our days.

Energy discharging can feel like a cold shudder or warm and tingly. You can assist this release by being aware of your body's endpoints. Three of these endpoints are your hands, feet and the crown of your head.

You are invited to explore waking up your endpoints. This can be done in a few short moments to encourage energy to flow more freely through you. Try them all for the experience. Then at any time when you notice yourself feeling stressed or emotional, you can use the ones you like best for on-the-spot support or relief.

Hands:

Shake out your arms and then wriggle your fingers, sensing the possibility of energy moving down through your arms and hands and out through your fingers. Use your opposite hand to sweep or wipe down your arms a few times from shoulder to fingertips, to awaken your awareness of each arm. You could also imagine light, colour or warmth streaming out of your fingertips to support the experience. How does this affect how you feel?

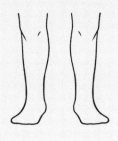

Feet:

To explore energy moving through your legs and out of your feet, shake out your legs, wriggle your toes and rotate your feet. Then place your feet flat and evenly on the ground. You can rub your feet on the ground, too (even if you have shoes on), to activate the nerve endings in the soles of your feet. Then sense the possibility of energy moving down through your hips and legs and out into the ground through your feet.

To enhance the effect, use your hands to brush downwards over your legs from hips down to feet, repeating a few times to awaken your awareness of your legs. When you get a chance you could also explore rubbing the soles of your bare feet on the ground to energise your feet. This works especially well on a textured surface like a carpet or grass. You can also imagine and feel into the possibility of receiving energy back up from the ground through your feet. Notice how this might support you and affect how you feel.

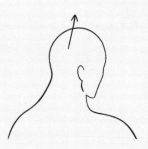

Crown:

Now imagine releasing energy upwards through your spine and out through the top of your head. Play with the idea of your spine being a hollow tube that allows energy to flow up and down through it. This can have an uplifting effect as you stand or sit taller, perhaps also helping you feel stronger in yourself. Try it out for a few moments with a focus on energy moving up through your spine, out through your crown and up into the sky. You can support the experience by wiping your hands up the back of your neck and head a few times. If you feel lightheaded at any point, you can place a hand on top of your head, which can help you to feel more grounded. Then you can focus on discharging energy through your hands or feet as an alternative. Play with these ideas, noticing how they affect your mind, body and mood.

As you experience life's ups and downs and different emotions, you might notice that opening the sense of energy being able to flow through and out of you can help you tolerate your feelings better, which is the basis for emotional resilience. Feel free to take this Mindful Body Moment any time to enhance your sense of personal strength and emotional flow. It can give your body and mind a quick energy boost, perhaps also boosting confidence in your ability to cope with whatever emotions might be moving through you at the time.

Another option for facilitating the flow and release of emotional energy is through the flow of energy between you and another person. This can also feel supportive and strengthening. When you feel emotional, it involves making contact with someone you feel close to, like calling them, or arranging to meet with them. This relationship-based channel for releasing emotional and nervous system energy receives dedicated attention in later chapters called 'Our Bodies Remember' and 'Healing Old Patterns, Enhancing Vitality'.

EXPLORING THE ENERGY OF DIFFERENT EMOTIONS

Anger: Presence plus power

Anger, with its lesser qualities of irritation and annoyance and its greater expression in rage, can offer empowerment. It makes you flex your muscles and gives you a surge of energy. Next time you feel it, let your body become it consciously. Grow, expand and strengthen your body as you stand tall and hold your head up high. Then take a deep breath and perhaps speak up while also considering how to use your power well. Anger helps you to stand strong in your views. Anger gives you the confidence and the ability to say 'No!' and 'Stop!', with conviction. To encourage you to use your power well and to avoid harming yourself or others, words like dignity, caring, and empathy, can guide you. Some simple questions to consider: What is really needed? Where do I need to set boundaries? What issue requires my assertiveness? How can I be powerful with heart?

Own your feelings and share with yourself or others what triggered the anger. You might say, 'I feel angry when ... happened, or when you said ...' instead of imposing views or judgements on others. It takes courage to share your feelings and express your needs. You might notice that your pulse races and your heart pounds. Doing this is an opening for others to share their perspectives and needs, too. If denied for too long, anger can collapse into helplessness. If you feel this way, look back in time for the first time you gave up on your ability to stand up for yourself. How can you claim back your power now?

Sadness: Presence plus soft tenderness

Sadness is a softening and melting into the vulnerability of being human, as opposed to bracing against it. With sadness also comes receptivity, such as being able to receive support and to be open to all your feelings – from love and joy through to pain and fear.

Sadness challenges you to be deeply touched and moved by life with its heartaches and exquisiteness. You are invited to open your heart to love and to also acknowledge the pain that can come when love is lost. Khalil Gibran adds a spiritual dimension by asking: 'God, please break my heart open so that I can let you in.' When you allow yourself to open and flow with sadness, when it appears, it will wash your hurts away and open you to a sense of life that is rich and deeply meaningful. It can also open you when the time is right to let love in. If you make a habit of not making space for sadness you might limit your ability to feel anything, including positive, delightful feelings. It is better to live with an open heart and to nurture sadness when it appears, than to live a cold, closed-off life.

Feeling your sadness can be beautiful for its own sake, such as when you allow yourself to be moved to tears by life's exquisite moments. Sadness can also point you to what you still might need to mourn, perhaps inviting you to make time to honor your feelings and how deeply you have loved. Most mourning will pass with time and there is some grief that never passes completely. The task then is, when the time is right, to make a special space inside your heart, where the one who you grieve for can live with you in spirit if they are no longer with you physically. This can be helpful as you find your way to go on living your life to the full.

Fear: Presence plus fixed focus

Fear is an alarm letting you know that something is dangerous or not right. Your body will freeze or leap into action and your instincts take over to protect you if you feel you are in danger. First you need to establish a place of safety and then act if you need to. If the threat amounts to nothing, and you find yourself still living in fear, more than you would like, then there is an acronym that might apply. It is 'FEAR': 'false evidence appearing real'. Your task is to use this alarm to discern what is real and what is not, or what is in the past and what is in the present. Worry and anxiety are examples of lingering fear. They linger because you either have not resolved something from your past or you have not had the courage to confront something in your present. Turning to your body instead of your thoughts and using self-soothing strategies like touch and breathing and perhaps adjusting your posture, can help you break a cycle of worrisome thinking. As fear begins to loosen its grip, emotions like sadness or anger might come to the fore. You can then channel the energy of these emotions to support you with tenderness or strength.

Note that, for some, tuning into feelings can be a smooth process. For others who have endured much suffering there can be resistance to looking inwards. It simply can feel too unsafe to touch into what is there. In cases of acute grief, trauma, chronic depression, anxiety or other psychiatric or medical conditions that can cause significant pain and distress, professional support is recommended.

Happiness: Presence plus a warming glow

Happiness can be anything from quiet contentment and joy through to leaps and bounds of excitement. How much are you able to embrace your happiness? Sometimes we restrict how much happiness we allow ourselves to feel, based on how people in our past have responded to our joy and excitability. Observe yourself next time you feel happy, and experiment with allowing your body to express even just a little bit more of it. Your creative juices might flow; your motivation might rise; you might become more social or playful. Play with how it feels and where it leads you.

Happiness is also a passing energy, just like all other emotions. In the words of Anais Nin, 'Life is a process of becoming, a combination of states we have to go through. Where people fail is that they wish to elect a state and remain in it.' The invitation is to embrace it all. This can give a state of underlying happiness as we come to trust and appreciate our emotional world. Life's ups and downs can also fuel inspiration, such as for the artists among us. Even non-artists might become bored without emotional variety. In the words of Salvador Dali, 'There are some days when I think I am going to die from an overdose of satisfaction.' It takes all of our emotional ups and downs to make life full, rich, interesting and meaningful.

Complex emotions

Feelings can overlay feelings and thoughts can overlay feelings, making your emotional world complex. For example, in depression you may need to confront suppressed feelings of anger, sadness and fear. Other complex feeling tones are jealousy, shame and guilt, which might contain elements of sadness (such as self-pity), fear (perhaps of not being good enough) and perhaps self-loathing (hating who and how you are and wishing you were different). Or perhaps you have gone against your own value system and simply need to find your way back. There are many emotional mixtures and permutations. When you can identify the basic ingredients in your emotional mix, you can consider the gifts of each one and address its needs one by one.

Or, if your emotions swing from very high to very low (this is called emotional lability) then your task is to find a middle ground to stabilise you. Perhaps you could explore the physical experience of your two emotional extremes and then physically feel into creating a middle ground in which you can feel more stable.

⇛ MINDFUL BODY PROCESS ⇚

Towards emotional insight and transformation

INTRODUCTORY WORDS

Engaging with our emotional world involves many internal and external conversations as we live in relationship with our feelings. This 'Mindful Body Process' offers a framework for engaging, particularly with our challenging feelings, in a constructive manner that supports neuroplasticity. Neuroplasticity is our brain's ability to be changed by external input, in this case towards our healing and emotional enrichment.

It is recommended to set aside at least 15 minutes for this process. It is a process that you can use to help you through times of emotional distress. It is also a process that you can use to work through age-old emotions by reconnecting with them in this guided way.

In this Mindful Body Process you are invited to acknowledge and name your emotions, scan back in time for triggers, invite a specific memory to focus on and intervene imaginatively in the outcome so it turns in your favour. Each step of the way you are encouraged to respond to emotional experience in supportive, empowering ways.

This process works because our emotional brain regions, that also store our emotional memories, are particularly suggestible and open to change or neuroplasticity. This change can literally re-pattern our brains so that when we recall an emotional memory that we have worked with, the interventions that we have used and the new outcome that we have imagined become fused together with the old memory. So, by re-entering a difficult memory we can turn it into a healing and nourishing experience, with imagination as our primary tool. Imagination can do this because of its close relationship with both emotions and memories. Both emotions and memories stir our imagination and are receptive to change via imaginative cues.

If your feelings on the day are positive, you can still explore this Mindful Body Process with an invitation to more thoroughly acknowledge and appreciate the positive. This can also promote positive brain change as you encourage yourself to remember and bask in your joys so that they can become a stronger part of your life.

THE PROCESS

How are you feeling? You might be feeling emotional now, which gives you material to explore. Or if your emotions are quiet and you wish to try out the process now, consider a feeling that you know well or that is recent enough that you can recall it easily. Maybe it is anxiety, depression, melancholy, irritation or anger, or a positive feeling like joy. Choose something that you are curious to learn more about. It can be helpful to write down your responses as you continue this exercise or you can simply respond spontaneously in your mind or talk them through with someone.

To start, focus on the feeling with you now or the feeling you would like to explore. Drop awareness into your body and take a few moments to notice how your feelings live inside you. You might notice particular parts of your body that capture your attention or how your posture shapes around your feelings. You might notice the quality of the feelings in your body or how they move inside you. Describe what you find the best way you can. You might feel tight, squeezed, fluttery, tingly, empty, sinking, aching, swirling, warm or anything else.

If you are struggling to identify the feelings in your body, just observe them for the time being and note where in your body you feel them most. You might feel a bit buzzy in your head, full of excitement all over, anxious in your chest and tight in your throat, tingly in your back, restless in your legs, numb, or heavy and tired. Describe whatever is really there for you. Already this process can take you out of the stories happening in your mind and into the feelings in your body in a more direct, visceral way.

Keep breathing naturally. Reminding yourself to breathe now and again can allow more space inside you for your emotional experience instead of holding your breath in fear or resistance.

How is your posture affected? If you were to give your current feeling and associated posture a name, what might it be? Perhaps one of the words you might use to describe this feeling could be excitable, agitated, scared or hysterical. Or you might choose to name it after an animal, like a roaring lion, an elephant, a fluttering butterfly or a timid mouse. Or you could name it after a film character, or simply a colour. There is no right and wrong, just what feels like a good fit and that can help you picture your feeling more clearly, and recall it easily, later. You can see this emotional state that you have just named, like a character that plays one role as part of the cast of characters that make up your life's emotional repertoire.

What are the kinds of thoughts and the state of mind that this character or this part of you is prone to? What are some of this character's beliefs about life?

Do any memories spring to mind that relate to you feeling this way? Spend a few moments allowing your mind to rewind through your associated memories. As you do this, consider what your earliest memory is of feeling this way. (Be spontaneous – maybe an age comes to mind, or a stage of life.) Reflect on this for a few moments.

You don't need to recall all the details, even just a sense of this memory is sufficient. You are now going to enter into this memory, explore it and perhaps intervene to affect the outcome.

Holding the memory in mind, notice where you are and who is with you. If you cannot pick up details, simply notice how you are feeling and see if you can get a hint of why you might be feeling this way. If you are able to pick up details, you might notice particular people, sounds, sights or smells around you. Fill in as many details as you can to help the moment come alive in your mind and body. What are you aware of? What is going on? And what is the trigger for your feelings?

If your experience is positive, such as remembering a time full of love, fun or joy, then there is no need to continue with the next steps of this process. Simply bask in the feelings that this memory brings.

If your memory is of an emotionally upsetting or distressing experience, then move on to consider this next step. It involves intervening in your memory to affect the outcome by inserting, for example, support or protection into your situation. To do so it is helpful to draw on imagination. You cannot change your past, but you can adjust your memories to include new, empowering elements based on your ability to intervene in your imagination now. This can allow shifts to your emotional world that can make a real difference to the quality of your life. Consider even something small that you can introduce with your imagination into the scenario. You might imagine bringing in someone who truly loves and supports you, from your current life. You could imagine them perhaps standing beside you in your memory and helping your younger self in some way, such as speaking up for you or taking you into their arms. This person might be someone in your life now or someone from your past. Or it might be a spiritual or holy figure or perhaps a superhero. Invite them in and notice how your body responds to their presence. From there, imagine watching the scene unfold like a movie in your mind, as you respond to their helpful intervention. In your imagination anything is possible, just like in your dreams. You can fly, magic is real, and anything can appear and disappear. Ask yourself as the movie unfolds, and as many times as you need to, 'What happens next?' 'What can I bring in next?' or 'What would be helpful now?' Each step of the way let the movie continue in your mind as you open to new and helpful people, things or scenarios. Keep the movie progressing in a positive direction towards a good outcome. Also, allow time for the scenes to play out in your mind and time for yourself, in your memory, to receive all the support you might feel that you need. For some this is a quick process, for others it can take longer. Feel into your body to help guide you to what is needed next. Continue with the process until you feel sufficiently taken care of. Continue until you like the final outcome.

Allow your body to grow into the feeling of this positive outcome. What part of your body draws your attention now? What is the feeling in that part and how are you feeling now, in general? This can help you to recall the feeling at a later time and it can reinforce your emotional transformation. Then take a deep breath, stretch, and find a posture that represents your good feelings. Perhaps place a hand supportively on your body or find a gesture that honors how you feel now. To mark the close of your exploration, hold your body position for a few moments while breathing naturally.

When you feel ready, move out into your day, making time if you wish, to write, draw, walk and think, or speak with someone about your process. This will help to consolidate it and allow you to move on. This is a process that you might use just once or you might choose to repeat it at other times towards insight and transformation of other memories and feelings. The choice is yours.

CHAPTER 6

Mindful Body Dreaming

*The biggest adventure you can ever take is to
live the life of your dreams.*

OPRAH WINFREY

Our mental images powerfully shape our bodies and our experience of life, predating our ability to think logically and to be intellectual. Children live in a sea of images with little distinction between what is 'real' and what is imagined. As adults we continue to inhabit, and be strongly influenced by, an image-rich internal world with, for example, all of our memories laden with images and associated feelings. These are also the dramas that show up in our dreams in their imagistic, symbolic and emotional ways. Growing our ability to be present and engage with the many moods and faces of our imagination and dreams can be an invaluable life skill for emotional healing and resilience. This chapter is dedicated to using the body as a tangible touchstone for navigating these explorations.

The main focus in this chapter is tackling your fears that can show up as nightmares. Once you acquire skills for working with your nightmares, these skills can be applied to any dreams or images from waking or sleeping life.

Working with images and dreams can help guide your life in inspiring, meaningful directions. The chapter ends by inviting you to visualise and embody a future that feels deeply aligned with your deepest dreaming self.

In these ways you are encouraged to spend time tuning into your imaginary, theta brainwave world. In so doing, you can discover a great source of self-awareness, healing, emotional resilience and inspiration. This is the world of Mindful Body Dreaming.

⇒ THE THETA HEALING POWER OF IMAGINATION ⇐

As mentioned in the previous chapter, our emotional brain regions are highly 'neuroplastic', or emotionally adaptable. In other words, our brains can be guided to change when we know how. We are perhaps wired this way because of the importance of emotional adaptability and learning to survive and thrive as a species in our communities and in our world.

Also, as touched on in the previous chapter, imagination, emotions and memory tend to follow each other. They all resonate in the theta brainwave frequency. Because of this connection, when we work with one of these areas, the others shift too. This is the reason why imagination can give us an effective way for creating desired change in our emotional world and in our memories. Thomas Budzynski, a biofeedback researcher, also points to the connection to learning. He describes the theta-, half-awake, half-asleep brainwave state as a transition zone in which we can absorb new information in an uncritical, non-analytical way. This is because images bypass our thinking brain's tendency towards assumptions and judgements that can limit our ability to change.

This chapter offers you more opportunities to play in the realm of imagination as a powerful tool for evolving and healing your emotions and memories.

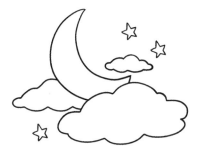

⇉ DREAMS MIRROR LIFE ⇇

It is helpful to consider that everyone and everything in your dreams reflect something of you in your waking life – as if calling out for your attention from the surreal world beneath your waking consciousness. Dreams are like a vast playing field for your sub-personalities and potentially a treasure chest full of useful advice. This is all contained in the images of the people, places and things that appear.

Useful questions to ask are: Why him? Why her? Why that? Why there? Why now? Rich material can emerge when you reflect on the qualities and feeling tones that you associate with these people, places and things, and consider how they might be relevant to you. This insight can help you deepen your self-awareness and enrich you in the process. You might gain insight into dynamics in your life that are not yet fully understood, or you might experience feelings that you know well. You might gain clarity about something in your emotional world or about how you view your circumstances. You might receive guidance. There are many possibilities.

THE 'AHA' FELT EXPERIENCE

How do you know with dream exploration that what you discover is helpful or true? The way to know is to feel how the images resonate with you. Jeremy Taylor, an expert group facilitator on dreams, and writer of books such as *Where People Fly and Water Runs Uphill*, refers to this as an 'aha experience'. It is a felt shift, such as a deep breath or a noticeable shift in your body when an insight about a dream truly hits home. So the only 'right' interpretation is the one that resonates with you and that feels right even if you cannot explain why.

⇉ SIX MINDFUL BODY DREAMING PROCESSES ⇇

For nightmares, deep fears and imagining new scenarios

Nightmares are confronting reminders of your deepest fears and can represent disowned or troubled parts of yourself. If you listen to and address what is reflected in your dreams about your life, you can experience big emotional shifts and impactful realisations. If you do not listen your nightmares may recur until you do heed the call.

Nightmares, particularly recurring ones, can also point to early life experience. For example, Sigmund Freud found that recurring dreams with a relatively unchanging structure often contain memory fragments of early traumas that could stem back even as far as the first years of life. With attention to the detail you can heal or find new ways to live with even very old feelings.

These six Mindful Body Dreaming Processes help the dreamer intervene in their dreams to create new, positive scenarios. They are intended for use while reflecting on your dream when awake. It can be helpful to write down your experience of engaging with your dreams. It can also be helpful to share your dream explorations with someone who knows you well. Because they know you well, their insight could prove helpful.

The first process invites you to connect with feeling safe and comfortable in yourself before you delve into your dream fears. This can support you in working with your fears. The four processes that follow, zoom in to opportunities for change in scary dreams. Each is designed to empower you. You might find that only one or two of the processes resonate with you. Play with them and use what works best for you. The sixth process, at the end of the chapter, offers an opportunity to visualise your future as you apply Mindful Body Dreaming to your values, goals and life choices.

⇉ MINDFUL BODY DREAMING PROCESS 1 ⇇

Finding feeling safe

As mentioned above, this process focuses on a safety point. It can be a helpful starting point when you are about to delve into your nightmares. You might actually have an image from your dream that feels wonderful and safe. You can recall this image now if it works for you. Or you can imagine that someone really caring and supportive is with you to accompany you on your journey into your dream. You could also call to mind a favourite place or use any image that evokes feelings of safety. Feel into your body where and how these feelings of safety live. Let the safe, perhaps heart-warming and soothing feelings grow, move and take shape inside you. What parts of your body do you notice most clearly? Perhaps associate a colour or an image to represent how you feel. You can also place your hand/s somewhere supportive on your body to anchor you to the feeling. Know that you can refer back to this image and feeling of safety whenever you feel you need to.

⇉ MINDFUL BODY DREAMING PROCESS 2 ⇇

Stepping into the role of a scary image to know it better

If your dream has a clear villain (such as an intruder or a chaser or other) or a scary scene, then this option may work for you. Imagine becoming this character or embodying qualities of the scary scene as if you are inside it. Take on a representative posture and mental attitude and feel into the perspective that it holds and what the motivations are of the scary character or scene. Describe it in detail – what it looks like and if it is a character, what it is wearing, how it sounds, and any other noteworthy details. By stepping into the scary role you are able to take over their threatening, terrifying hold over you. Instead, you can become them. Be curious about why they are the way they are. Reflect on how the dream image might be a mirror for some aspect of your life, such as by asking 'Why him or her or this, now?' This might indicate something in your life that feels threatening or terrifying.

Case study 6: A core issue reframed – Sandy's nightmare

Sandy experienced a terrifying recurring dream that had begun in her childhood. In her dream she was a small fish in a deep pool of water with many black fish furiously circling around her. In analysing the dream, she first explored becoming the little fish. She felt trapped by the ominous black fish. She also felt terrified about what would happen to the innocent-looking deer standing just ahead on the embankment in her dream. There is a raging fire approaching the deer from a forest behind. Sandy, as the little fish, desperately wants to save the deer, but she can't. This impotence in the dream left Sandy feeling panicked, which was a familiar feeling in her life.

In waking life, Sandy was depressed and worried excessively about others. When her symptoms of depression were strong, she cried a lot, which led others to worry about her. This only compounded Sandy's worries. Sandy had grown up in a single-parent family and she felt responsible for her mum. She felt like she was her mother's whole world. In her dream she associated the deer with her mother. She described the deer as vulnerable and in need of protection. In waking life she experienced her mother as emotionally vulnerable even though her mother is a strong personality who is not afraid to speak her mind.

We explored Sandy's dream images one by one. I encouraged her to get up and move around the room as much as she felt comfortable in a manner representative of the image that we were exploring. I stood up and moved with her for my own insights or ideas about her experience and to help her feel more comfortable with moving. When Sandy stepped into being the scary, circling black fish, to feel into their perspective, it dawned on her that these fish were not trying to torment the little fish. They were actually being fiercely protective! They needed to swim around furiously because of how desperately the little fish wanted to leap out to save the deer, which Sandy could now see was ridiculous. The black fish held the perspective that doing so would only lead to the little fish's death.

This realisation had an enormous impact on Sandy. How could that be? It changed her experience of her dream completely. The black fish were in fact wiser than the little fish. This reminded her of how her mother is fiercely protective of her at times, too. It also reminded her of how fiercely protective she can feel towards her mother, based on a belief that her mother really needs that emotional support. What if Sandy did not need to fear the fish at all? What if, instead of fearing the black fish, she should listen to them? This realisation changed everything. It reframed the way Sandy related to her dream and it changed something deep inside of her that had previously seen protective fierceness as a destructive force, as opposed to a constructive one. In our discussions that followed she turned from feeling terrified and panicked in relation to the dream and in relation to her role in her family, to starting to really hear that it is not her place to 'save' her mother (represented in her dream by the deer). She realised that feeling so fiercely protective can also be a noble quality. We also considered what it could offer her to apply some of this noble energy to her depression. It gave her inner strength that helped her stand taller and to see her protective instinct as a good quality. She came to view her depression as representing a younger, confused version of herself that needed guidance. Contacting her inner strength felt reassuring and empowering for Sandy as she sensed her ability to step into this new and mature perspective.

⇒ MINDFUL BODY DREAMING PROCESS 3 ⇐

Imagining your own ending

In this process you creatively evolve your dream images in positive directions to access the personal empowerment that they can give you. Imagination and visualisation are your tools. Start with the images that you remember from your dream and, from there, play with possibilities in the surreal. Not only can this be helpful for shifting your experience of your dreams, it can also be a great problem-solving tool for applying to anything in your life. It can be a fun process and one that works really well with children, helping them to understand their dreams and apply this understanding to life's challenges.

Sandy's nightmare continued

As part of Sandy's dream reflections, she identified water as an element that really resonates with her. In identifying this, she wondered if water could indicate something about her true nature. I invited her to play in her imagination with some ideas. I first asked her to imagine being immersed in water and adopt the movement of being or swimming in water. After a few moments of quiet, Sandy shared that she always felt at peace when she was around or in water. When feeling this way it reminded her of how deeply she cared for her special people. It also reminded her of qualities that she felt came naturally to her, such as patience and creative flow. She loved painting and described it as her favourite way to express her creativity. I asked her to think of the little fish from her dream in a new light, without the black fish circling it. I also asked her to imagine the scene without the fire in the distance. How would the little fish feel simply to be in the water? She replied that the fish could now enjoy swimming around in the water instead of trying to leap out of it.

As part of this process, Sandy felt that she needed to give the fish permission to stay in the water. Applying imagination proactively again, she imagined re-entering her dream to give the fish permission to stop trying to 'save' the deer. This took shape as a conversation between the fish and herself. She identified the little fish as a goldfish. As the fish, she relaxed and allowed herself to sink into her deep waters and to have permission to explore her watery home. She could now be free to find some goldfish friends (instead of the black fish) to be with and play with. This brought new-found joy with soft smiles of amazement and relief. We spent some time feeling into this experience in her body, filling her body with a sense of connectedness with her watery, peaceful and possibly playful nature, too. Sandy spoke about feeling more trusting in this space. In her waking life she knew that she wanted to become an art teacher and that she would do all that she could to realise this dream. For now, though, she was content to breathe a sense of trust and warm community with like-minded 'fish' through her body. Her whole demeanor softened and her voice sounded more song-like as she relaxed into this experience.

She ended the session feeling grateful for the permission to rest into her true nature instead of trying to be someone else. We reflected on the contrast to her tendency to throw herself 'out of the water' to take care of others at her own expense. She could now be more aware of this tendency and invite herself back into her soft, fluid sense of self and belonging in her element when she caught herself 'out of the water'. We spoke about how she could still care for others, but in a balanced way, whereby she also took care of her own needs. Noticing her breathing became a reference point that she could draw on whenever she needed to, for diving back into her watery nature.

She related this to her work choices, speaking of how she had spent her early twenties exploring different work options. Now in her late twenties she decided to return to study fine arts so that she could pursue her dream of teaching art to adolescents. This was a scary path as she went from being financially independent to wondering how she would be able to make ends meet as an art student. She also wondered whether she would find a teaching position in the kind of school that she dreamed of working in. Essentially she wondered how she would be able to survive in her 'element'. Through the experience of imagining herself in water, and feeling how supportive the quality of it felt to her, however, she was confident that no matter how difficult the path would be, she needed to follow it.

I felt that her dream transformation would not be complete until she also took care of the deer. In order to build on the realisation that it is not her place to save her mother, I invited her to again use her proactive imagination. I felt that this would consolidate her new sense of self. Sandy chose to imagine the deer reaching safety. She envisioned the deer running and running until it reached a safe haven far away from the flames, with a community of other warm and welcoming deer. She connected this to a sense of trust that her mother can be supported by other people, particularly Sandy's aunt. She also knew that her mother would not want Sandy to feel like she needed to protect her, so she knew her thinking was based on a false belief. With this in mind, she could relax more deeply into being herself, as the goldfish in her own waters, with the deer now safe and cared for.

On completing her art course, Sandy interviewed for her ideal art-teaching job and got the position. Her depression still rears its head occasionally, as does her pattern of over-extending herself for others. But her sense of self has become stronger and she feels more skilled in dealing with her feelings. This allows her to recover more quickly than before and it reduces the intensity of her symptoms. She also has become more motivated to take care of herself. This included going on a course of antidepressant medication, for the short term, to help take the edge off her condition, and to help her experience life differently. We all have good days and bad days. These may continue even after big realisations from exploring dreams. The most important marker is that there is improvement in how we feel as we heed the advice that we receive from exploring our dreams. For Sandy this is certainly proving to be the case.

⇒ MINDFUL BODY DREAMING PROCESS 4 ⇐

Linking dream images with the day before

According to the psychiatrist and physician-turned-dream-worker, Montague Ullman, dreams are often influenced by what happened the day before. Looking at how we can connect dreams to events in recent waking life can shift the emotional charge from your dream to the matter in your life that needs attention. This can be used as impetus to seek practical solutions to your challenges.

Case study 7: Sam's dream

A friend of mine, Sam, dreamed of being on a beach. He looked down and was shocked to discover a deep gash on his right knee. In his dream he couldn't remember how it had happened. The next dream clip was of him being in a doctor's room and agreeing to have his right leg amputated. The final dream clip was waking in a hospital bed to discover his right leg had been amputated. A state of absolute shock and horror exploded in him. On waking up from the dream he was elated to discover that his leg was still there!

Sam had recently started a new job and was experiencing difficulty communicating with one of his superiors. He described her as an outwardly strong yet inwardly insecure woman, who perhaps felt challenged by Sam's strong personality and confidence. Because of her status in the business, Sam feared that she could compromise his reputation in his new job. After a confrontation with her early in the week, Sam asked for a meeting to try and clear the air. The meeting was scheduled for later that same week on the Friday afternoon. Sam's dream appeared on the Thursday night before. Thursday had been a day filled with high anxiety about the meeting. Sam called me on Friday morning to ask if I had time to hear his dream, and if I could offer him any ideas that might be helpful. Sam associated the dream with his anxiety at work. It felt crucial that he be able to prove his abilities at work as he was still on a probation period. Cutting off his right leg could represent his progress being amputated by this woman.

Dreams tend to reflect compelling feelings that can relate to the day before and that can also cast a long shadow back in time, which can be helpful to study. In Sam's case,

I knew that his feeling restricted by an intimidating superior cast a long shadow back to his childhood when he had often felt intimidated, restricted and thrown off balance by his father. When I reminded him of this, Sam quickly realised that facing these feelings in his current work life could be an opportunity for him to engage with his feelings differently. He reminded himself of how far he had come since childhood, in building up his self-confidence, and he aspired to use his confidence respectfully in contrast to his father's emotionally abusive style. He was aware that people in positions of authority, who showed even a hint of disrespect or 'emotional abuse' towards him, were a trigger. At these times he instantly regressed to feeling helpless and hopeless again, giving all of his power away to the other person. He knew that his father was in charge when he was a child, but now, as an adult, he needed to remind himself that he was in charge of his life and that even with his superior at work he could remain respectfully confident in a way that felt empowering. I invited him to feel the quality of respectful confidence in his body and to stand in a posture that he felt represented this attitude. He planned to remind himself of this attitude before his meeting later that day.

The meeting went well. Sam and his co-worker listened to each other and she appreciated how he reached out to her to open their communication and resolve their issues. She actually had not seen an issue to the extent that he had, and was only aware of one difference of opinion, which they eventually resolved. It was an excellent day at work for the rest of the day, too. This was him standing firmly on his two legs and feet, feeling strong and warmly respectful – an inspiring, energising stance.

In the book *Mindsight*, author Daniel Siegel says that dreaming is 'one of the important ways we integrate memory and emotion,' with dreams serving as 'an amalgam of memories in search of resolution.' For this reason it is helpful to start with the feeling tone of the dream, which may be associated with many memories clustered together. This was the case with Sam's feelings. The dream reminded him of how he had felt growing up with his father, which reinforced his reactions to others in positions of authority.

So when next you have a dream, you might consider what happened the day before and how this might remind you of your past experience, too. Also, consider what is really needed now. From there, listen inwards and be open to what comes.

⇒ MINDFUL BODY DREAMING PROCESS 5 ⇐

Looking for empowering possibilities in imagination and dreams

In Process 5 you look for empowering, helpful elements within your dream that you might not initially be aware of. The task is to look into the images in their context and attempt to identify supportive or empowering elements that we might not have noticed before.

Sam's dream exploration continued

During another conversation at a later date, we revisited Sam's dream. After our previous conversation in which Sam shared his dream, it struck me that he had given permission for his leg to be amputated. I was curious to ask him about this and to consider how he might respond differently if he had felt more empowered. He was happy to reflect on it. He shared that he had not thought twice about giving permission. He had not focused on it because of the shock of the next scene in which his leg was missing. This clearly was a place in his dream where he could explore responding differently to affect the outcome. It was perhaps where he could take back his power in his dream world to affect how he felt in his waking life.

At my encouragement, he actively imagined a new scenario. He said 'No' to the doctor, 'my leg can be saved'. Then he imagined waking up to his leg still in place and healed. A wonderful feeling tingled down his right leg. On standing up, he at first felt tentative, then stronger, more grounded, and steady on his two legs. Because of this experience he felt stronger and more physically grounded, which perhaps helped him with future encounters with people who might intimidate him.

Reflecting back again on how he gave permission to the doctor in his dream, he wondered how this might apply to his relationship with the woman at work. He wondered if he had somehow given unwitting permission to her, or reason, to stunt his progress. With the doctor in his dream Sam had felt that it was inevitable that his leg needed to be cut off. But was it really inevitable that the woman at work cut off his potential for progress? Their meeting to clear the air had gone well, so maybe his fears were unfounded. Sam was aware now of his two legs standing strongly and firmly on the ground. This helped him to feel more confident in his abilities, and able to focus at work.

These moments become reference points that we can draw on over time. This was especially important for Sam because, some time after his dream, his challenges with this person surfaced again and their personalities clashed. His challenge was to remind himself of his dream insights and to practise standing into his own respectful authority. Old wounds can take a while, and lots of practise, to heal. Our task is to reduce the impact of these wounds on our lives so that we can feel more empowered and fulfilled.

Case study 8: Mandy's dream

Finding something empowering inside of your dream may not be as clear as answering a question differently (like in Sam's dream). You may need to consider your dream closely to find empowering elements. In Mandy's dream she is sitting in a classroom and feels full of self-pity in contrast to a friend who she feels envious of, who is sitting in front of her. The woman that she envies seems confident and sits in an athletically strong and flexible manner with legs folded under her on a chair and appearing very comfortable in her body.

Reflecting on the dream, Mandy scans through the details to try to find something empowering. What she finds is the classroom setting. This, in her words, is her 'success space' such as at school and university. She also realises that the woman who she envies is non-academic, so it dawns on her that this woman, in waking life, probably would not feel accomplished in a classroom setting.

On being invited to do so, Mandy grows the image of the classroom in her imagination and in her body's feelings. She describes feeling big, contained and proud and able to contain her feelings of self-pity in a nurturing way. In this way Mandy combined the bigger, helpful traits associated with the 'classroom', with her feeling small and sorry for herself. This helped her to transfer her feelings of success to being able to hold herself through her difficult emotions.

I invited her to give her self-pitying self some advice from the perspective of the 'classroom'. It went something like this: 'When you are feeling jealous and pitiful, remember your talents. Let this remind you that you have a lot to be proud of. Going more regularly to the gym will help, too, so that you too can be fitter and more flexible in your body, like your friend is in her body.' A practical action plan came out of exploring this dream. She worked towards investing in feeling better about herself, to pity herself less and become more comfortable in her own skin.

MONITOR CHANGE IN WAKING AND DREAMING LIFE

As time goes by, notice how your dreams might change and what themes may need further attention. For example, when healing trauma, dreams may gradually become less frightening. You might start to see themes from the scary, old recurring dream, but with new positive elements appearing such as relating to feeling less or no longer threatened. So your process can gradually evolve to incorporate more and more of your new life themes and experiences.

Also be curious about changes in your waking life as you play with new images and possibilities. To get a sense of your progress, you might reflect on your life some years ago and compare it to now. How have you changed? What might you have learned along the way that has improved the quality of your life? You might also notice that some old themes still continue to surface. Life is a journey. Your task is to engage with your emotions as you feel ready to do so and know that you can create changes to positively influence the quality of your life.

Change is also not linear and finite. Change cycles as we re-experience old feelings, consolidate new awarenesses and evolve new possibilities. Progress may need reinforcement and repetition of lessons as we grow and develop. If it feels like a slow process, recognising the areas of our lives where change has really happened can be encouraging. Even if old themes resurface every now and again, we probably deal with them differently now and our learning today can help us to deal with the challenges we might face tomorrow.

DREAMING OF DEATH

One of the scariest dreams is about death. Stepping into the world of something that terrifies you allows you to become curious about the dream's story. Some questions that you might consider include: 'What could this represent in my life?' 'What in my life might need to die, in order for something new to be born, or for me to open to a new path?' Look out for the qualities of the person or thing that dies. These can provide clues. If in your dream a child dies, it might represent a young and vulnerable part of you that you need to let go of. If it is someone old, it might mean releasing an old, outmoded way of being. If your death image is accompanied by other people, places or things, how do you feel about these particular people, places or things in your waking life? What about them is connected with a part of you that you need to let go of or evolve at this time? If it is you who dies in a dream then it might point to the need for personal change. It is unusual to dream of yourself dying unless there has been trauma in your past that still feels threatening. If it does come up, it might point to trauma resolution that is still needed. The metaphor of 'What in my life needs to move out so something new can move in?' can be helpful.

Be open to your associations and play with meanings until one feels right. According to the dream expert Jeremy Taylor, no matter how death might appear in our dreams, it is always associated with our personal growth and development. When we can see and accept this, it can lead to an equally powerful experience of rebirth.

TOWARDS WHOLENESS

Carl Jung believed that dreams represent a drive towards growth and wholeness. Dreams do so by holding up a mirror, showing us what really is going on in our emotional world or qualities that we might not be focusing on. These might be parts of us that are deemed unacceptable or that we might deny or project onto others. For example, a stoic, unemotional man might see himself sobbing in a dream that reflects his lost emotions. According to Jung, in order to feel whole we need to own the feelings that show up in our dreams. For example, the sobbing man in his dream might be showing the dreamer that his emotions need to be consciously felt and expressed in order to achieve personal growth and a sense of wholeness. In this way our dreams can help us tap into deep and hidden potential that we can then integrate into our lives.

With such a valuable resource in our imagination and dreams, we might want to take full advantage of it in proactive ways. As explored in this chapter and the chapter before, we can re-transcribe memories by intervening imaginatively in our dreams. We can also ask for dream guidance by seeding our minds with a question about an issue, doing so as we relax before drifting off to sleep and then taking note of our dreams as soon as we wake. Imagination can also be a great tool for creative brainstorming while awake, to help us explore possible solutions to any of life's challenges. There are many possibilities. And sometimes just 'sleeping on it' can bring relief to our problems by allowing our brainwaves to shift our perspectives naturally as we drift off and return from deeper, dreamier realms.

MYSTERY AND EMOTIONAL HEALING

Dreams can be a goldmine for psychological excavation and on some level they also remain a mystery with a purpose that might be beyond interpretation. There is a time for seeking meaning from our dreams and there is a time for embracing the mystery.

Fortunately, the simple act of spending time with our dream images can be a powerful tool for emotional healing. When we focus on our dream images they can bring stillness to linear time. This stilling, according to Gerald Epstein, author of *Waking Dream Therapy*, is required 'to effect healing of man's emotional suffering'. In other words, simply spending time with our dreams and imagination can offer welcome relief from the pace and demands of a busy life. Whether applied to understanding our lives or to simply appreciating our dream world for what it is, our dreams and imagination can tune us in to a vast and wondrous internal world of resources and enrichment.

⇒ MINDFUL BODY DREAMING PROCESS 6 ⇐

Visualising your future

Here is an opportunity to apply imagination to service your future. It is an invitation to visualise how you would love your life to look ten years from now and then work backwards to the present, to align your life with your long-term vision.

To start, let yourself imagine your ideal life ten years from now. You might like to write down what you think of, to keep track of the process. Visualise areas of your life such as relationships, family, money, career and social contribution, travel, studies, spirituality, friends, home, mentors and supportive community – anything you can think of. You can even draw a picture representing these ideas, such as drawing your ideal home. Allow your mind and imagination complete freedom. Along with considering how to fill your life with joy and how to apply your talents in meaningful ways, it is important to also consider your life legacy and the kind of contribution you would like to make in our world.

Then consider how your life would look five years from now in relation to your ten-year vision. What would you need to be doing or have started by then? And what would characterise you as a person aligned with this long-term vision? Then consider the same for two years from now. What is happening and how are you living? What steps could you take one year from now, and in your present life, to begin setting something in motion, even something very small, towards your inspiring vision?

How does your body feel as you consider this? What characterises the person you become when you align with your life vision? How do you stand, think, feel and relate to your dreams? Come up with an image or a word to describe yourself and to help you recall the feelings more easily. Choose what feels most inspiring and enlivening. Write it down or draw it if you wish, to help you remember it.

Once you have your vision and an idea of your long- and short-term goals in relation to it, then all that is left to do is act on it. Your actions are what will keep your vision alive. A good attitude to also carry with you is one of trusting in the process of life. Along with your vision and actions, it is also important to read the signposts along the way and trust that when one door closes another door opens. Perhaps this can remind us all to follow not only our heads for guidance, but also our hearts, our intuition, and life itself, that can have a wisdom and timing all of its own.

CHAPTER 7

Our Bodies Remember

The body remembers, the bones remember, the joints remember,
even the little finger remembers. Memory is lodged in pictures and
feelings in the cells themselves. Like a sponge filled with water,
anywhere the flesh is pressed, wrung, even touched lightly, a
memory may flow out in a stream.

CLARISSA PINKOLA ESTES

⇒ OUR BODIES REMEMBER EVEN
THE FIRST YEAR OF LIFE ⇐

I am lying with my body and head completely covered by a blanket. I am so cozy and warm that I could stay here for a long while. I am waiting for the teacher to ask us to emerge from our blankets. Then I hear the invitation to come out when I feel ready. I know I have to come out at some point, because that is the instruction, although I don't feel like it. I slowly lift one side. Then, before I have time to think about it I have removed the blanket and burst out into the open. I sit with eyes open, adjusting to the light and feeling a bit dazed. I look around the room to the other bundles of people wrapped in blankets, moving and emerging in their own time.

This was an activity as part of my course on Somatic Psychology. The focus of the exercise was on connecting with the possibility that our bodies remember all of life's experiences in a felt, embodied way, and that re-enacting our birth experience evokes the tone of the experience as it really was at the time. I was not sure what to make of it, at that time. Later, when we had an opportunity to share, we were asked if something about this experience felt familiar in relation to our lives or how we navigate life's transitions. With some reflection I could relate to a pattern of fluctuating between times of dreamy inner peace, taking life slowly while feeling quietly in control, and times of startle or anxiety. I know these feelings well. The anxiety reminded me of when I get triggered by interactions with the outside world, such as feeling rushed or when I feel intimidated by people with strong, assertive personalities. It is as if in those moments I lose touch with my own intellect and instincts as I look outside myself for what to do or say next. This can make me go mentally blank and fumble for words as I shrink inside myself.

We were asked to find out from our parents, if possible, what our actual birth was like. When we returned to share with the class, I heard many stories of how people's actual birth experiences correlated with their feelings and behaviour when enacting the birth process from under a blanket. In my story, I learned that I was induced after many hours of a natural birth process that did not progress as it should have. On researching the effects of induction medication, I learned that the experience is that of speeding up contractions so that there is no sense of the mother's body having its own rhythm. So a baby, I imagine, would also feel at the mercy of these fast and chaotic labour rhythms leading up to birth. Perhaps this explains my anxiety or sudden sense of feeling overwhelmed when I am rushed, out of control or at the mercy of external forces, including people I find intimidating.

I could identify with all of this deeply. Over the years I have developed a tendency to be very well prepared for what I need to be, which helps me to counteract an anxious sense of falling behind. For example, I used to complete school or university assignments ahead of schedule for fear of not completing them in time. And the trigger is still there to this day when I do not plan ahead, even for small daily tasks. This may be leaving the house on time to take children to school, which otherwise can easily turn into some degree of frenzy. A fear of being late fuels this rushing around and raises my anxiety levels. Gaining great physical control through many years of being a ballet dancer, and then a Yoga practitioner, has also helped me to curtail a deep fear of feeling out of control. It has helped me to build self-control and greater self-worth into my body. I am also better able to breathe and feel my way through triggering times, with compassion for my process, even though I still do need to remind myself now and again that I am in charge of my responses now.

Could this anxiety and startle response, when feeling that others or circumstances have power over me, stem from my birth experience? I might never know for sure. What I do know is that the exercise in class that day evoked an 'aha' moment, which resonated deeply with me as I experienced those familiar feelings.

During my years of study I made a personal choice to see a psychologist who works in a body-inclusive way. My therapist allowed me to stay under the blanket for many sessions until I felt ready to emerge in my own way and in my own time. Something inside of me let go to allow greater relaxation into my body. I allowed myself to feel that I had permission to have my own timing and that I did not need to be rushed. This permission felt, and still feels, empowering when I recall it. In my life at the time, and even to this day, I invite myself to prepare and not feel rushed so that timing can simply be structure for life rather than something threatening. Especially with such deeply ingrained experiences, anxiety can still surface years afterwards –

in my case in my reaction to feeling rushed. A more relaxed experience to juxtapose it with, can help. Another insight also dawned on me from this experience – about permission for me to trust my inner knowing more as a guide for my life, instead of feeling guilty as if I should be living a different life according to standards I imagine that others have.

Another physical re-enactment of a stage of child development that led to an 'aha' moment for me, was when we were crawling and exploring making our way up to standing. I felt cautious, initially, and found myself wanting to stand up slowly. Then, as I stood up, I felt strangely triumphant as I planted my two feet firmly on the ground. My mother had told me that my sister, who is a year and a half older than me, had been jealous of the attention that I received when I first started to walk. She acted out by pushing me over repeatedly in my early walking attempts. This led to my crawling for many months more. When I did finally stand up again I must have been determined to be as steady as possible to counter her attempts to push me over.

I remember seeing a photo of myself when I was around 18 months old. In the photo I am standing, looking very balanced on my two little legs, facing the camera squarely with a smile on my face and a banana in my hand. To me it looks like I am a little cowboy, steady and ready for anything, with a 'banana' gun in my hand, as if to say, 'Don't mess with me.' What I had never consciously noticed as an adult, was my body memory of this.

As a dancer later in life I was complimented for my good balance and for being assured on my legs. I feel a connection between this and the steadiness I grew from having to watch out for my sister in my first experience of standing. I am also to this day nervous of walking down steep hills, which may also be a subconscious residue from being repeatedly pushed over.

From a somatic psychology perspective you could explore any stage of child development to evoke the tone of the experience that you had when you first developed the ability, such as to crawl or walk or stand. We are also changed by our experiences later in life, but it's the very early years that leave the most enduring imprint.

MUMMY AND I ARE ONE

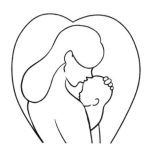

Another example of the power of pre-verbal, early life memory is found in the primal connection that we all seem to have with 'Mummy'. Dr Lloyd Silverman, a pioneer in the therapeutic application of subliminal messages, discovered one simple five-word sentence that apparently has universal effects when delivered subliminally (as opposed to being told to us when we listen consciously). 'Mummy and I are one.'

This sentence became the subject of hundreds of subliminal research projects and has proven effective with programs for weight loss, smoking cessation, alcoholism, academic achievement and other applications. Subliminal messages are picked up by our brain's theta, dreaming brainwave state, which taps into our emotional brain regions and our emotional memories. This is what is thought to make subliminal messages so effective – they can cut through critical thinking processes to access emotional memories and deep longings directly. These emotional memories begin recording as soon as we become conscious of our experience. This consciousness is believed to be in place in utero at a time when we literally were 'one with Mummy', carried in her womb and immersed in her world.

What is it about the words 'Mummy and I are one' that has such a powerful effect? Dr Silverman believes that these words represent a symbiotic fantasy of an archetypal experience of merging with an ideal mother figure. The result is an experience available to all of us, of deep, inner peace, and connection with something bigger. It is carried within us, generally on a subconscious level, throughout life.

From a psychological point of view it can be a subconscious yearning to return to the safety and comfort of the womb. The womb can represent a blissful, warm and containing space before the pain of birth and inevitable separation from 'Mummy' as we grow older. It can represent the space before encountering all the anxieties and responsibilities of independent living. For some, the experience in utero could have been stressful, such as if the mother lived an unhealthy lifestyle or was chronically stressed, which both can affect the fetus. According to Dr Thomas Verny, a leading authority on the effects of prenatal environment on personality development, everything a pregnant mother feels and thinks is communicated through neurohormones to her unborn child as surely as alcohol and nicotine are. Even if the gestation period included stress, 'Mummy and I are one' seems to remain a yearning for a blissful union.

YOUR RELATIONSHIPS

Relationships are an arena where the yearning for blissful union can play out. When we initially meet a romantic partner, for example, it is common to project onto them the hope of filling a 'Mummy and I are one' sized hole in our psyche. It is usually the case that with such high expectations we end up disappointed – relationships are complex and we all have our ups and downs. It is possible in long-term relationships to work towards an ultimate kind of bliss, although it does take commitment and conscious loving from both people to know each other's hurts and to hold and respond to each other with loving care. It also requires acceptance that nobody is perfect, and a desire to learn from times of discord.

From a spiritual point of view, the yearning for oneness has been associated with a mythical loss of paradise. Spirituality can also offer a remedy for this longing for 'oneness' through spiritual or religious practice.

Once acknowledged and owned for what it is, perhaps consciously visualised as a positive, nourishing space, and perhaps cultivated through spiritual practice, our primal yearning for 'Mummy and I are one' can offer us gifts. Gifts can include abiding inner peace that we can choose to carry with us consciously through life, with origins deep inside our body memory.

⇒ MINDFUL BODY MOMENT ⇐

Visualising comfort and warm support for building inner peace

Our inner peace is so closely intertwined with how we felt welcomed, held and responded to in our earliest years. Allowing ourselves to imagine an ideal mother figure or any other image, if we prefer, that helps us to feel warmly soothed, can remind us of an inner peace we might have experienced in utero and that we can recreate in our felt experience now. Spiritual or religious practice, as well as spending time in nature, can serve this function, too, allowing a wave of peace to grow from deep inside us and soothe our souls.

To help you reconnect with feelings of comfort and inner peace at any time you might wish to, you can use this Mindful Body Moment.

Imagine who or what might represent loving care and support for you. You might imagine an ideal mother figure, for example. For some this might be your actual mother, who you have a nourishing relationship with. For others, you might choose the image of someone else you know or it could be based on an image you might have seen, perhaps in a film or in a book, that represents the qualities for you of comfort and support with a warm, soothing presence. Some might wish to choose a meaningful spiritual figure or some might choose to imagine a favourite beautiful scene in nature that feels soothing and supportive. Call on your image to be with you now. Notice how your image of choice arrives and how it shifts your feelings. Let its presence grow to feel strong and warm.

Soak up the feelings. Breathe them into and through you, allowing the feelings to seep into your body as much as you can. Even if you can only allow a little bit in, let that little bit feed you. You might imagine what your life could feel like if this warm, soothing presence was with you more often. How might this make your life different? Stay with the feelings and consider if there is a part of your body where the experience seems more noticeable, such as in your heart area or your arms. If you find a place, focus there for a few moments, perhaps breathing into the area and exploring it with some movement or touch so that you can sense it more clearly. To finish this process, think of a way to incorporate it into your posture to help you carry the experience forward into your day. Once you have found a posture, stay and breathe with the experience for a few more moments to really give it time to register in your brain and being. Then, as you feel ready, move back out into your day.

⇒ 'REMEMBERING' SO FAR BACK ⇐

If you try to remember your first year of life, you will most probably draw a blank. This is because we tend to look for an explicit storyline or to recall the factual details or chronological events of our lives. But if you enquire through the feelings in your body, by re-enacting developmental stages connected to different times in your life, and use cues like imagination to call on these different times, your body will likely reveal the quality of your experience. This involves accessing your implicit memory bank as your non-verbal, physical and feeling-based record of life.

TRY IT OUT

Imagine being held as a baby, resting in your mother's arms. How do you feel? Is your breathing easy and full? Do you feel warm inside and safe? Or does your breath quicken and your body tense? Your experience is what is true for you. Whether or not you can corroborate your experience with what actually happened, your experience remains true because it feels true. This experience can tap into a very early imprint around your ability to relax, and to trust that you will be taken care of. What is your relationship with relaxation and trusting the support of others? Or perhaps you feel you need to go it all alone and because of this you carry a knot of tension deep down in your core?

As another opportunity to explore your implicit, feeling-based memory, simply say the word 'No'. This word can show you something about your relationship with assertiveness. Say 'No' again and notice what happens in your throat and in your body. Do you feel strong and grounded in your 'No'? Or do you feel suppressed or stopped somehow? Where do you feel this in your body? We begin to explore saying 'No' from around two years old, which is a time when patterns relating to saying 'No', and how people around us responded, can be set in place. Later in life we might consciously work through difficulties we may experience with saying 'No'. This can translate into our ability to set boundaries, respect limits and stand up for what we believe in. What does your 'No' feel like today? Do you tend to have a very strong 'No'? Or is yours meek and mild? Both have stories to tell about how you were influenced in your formative relationships.

These are two examples of implicit memory at work. With awareness, it is this level of our experience that we can learn to work with to bring about deep and meaningful shifts in our sense of self, our relationships and our lives. The Mindful Body Process for emotional insight and transformation, in the emotions chapter, can be useful in working through early, implicit memories, too. So if you noticed your 'No' is not as clear as you would like it to be, or your sense of safety in your mother's arms was not as warm and welcoming as it could have been, you can explore it further and insert resources to assist your younger self. This can allow you to shift feelings you might have carried with you for as long as you can remember, towards experiencing life differently.

⇒ BLUEPRINTS FROM THE FIRST YEARS OF LIFE ⇐

Following birth we open to a whole new world. How we are received in our parent's or caretaker's arms ideally recreates something of the warm, blissful oneness of the womb. Words like inner peace, basic trust and sense of security are used by theorists, and describe the healthy outcome of our first year transitioning into the world of air and family. Anxiety, mistrust and insecurity are also possible as outcomes if our first years are lacking the love, consistency and nurturing that babies need. Insecurity can also result when factors besides our parents interfere with the ability to form secure attachment, such as medical interventions that may remove baby from parents out of necessity. Or perhaps a parent has unresolved trauma that stands in their way. Our relative security and insecurity can affect us in many ways including our ability to feel contained, stable and emotionally fulfilled.

FEELING SECURE OR INSECURE

A theory that delves deeply into the early formation of feeling secure or insecure is Attachment Theory. The term *Attachment* in this sense refers to the deep and enduring connection established between a baby and their primary caregiver, mainly in the first year of life. Attachment Theory considers the child's perspective in terms of how safe, trusting and secure they feel, based on their parent's responsiveness. In turn, this affects the child's expectations that the world is either a safe or dangerous place. Later in life an original attachment pattern can either be reinforced or changed, depending on the nature of later relationships.

To investigate Attachment Theory, developmental psychologist Mary Ainsworth carried out foundational research many years ago. She looked at specific patterns in infant and toddler behaviour when placed in what she called a Strange Situation. The Strange Situation was designed to create some distress when the children were separated from their mother, and then re-introduce the mother and observe the child's reactions. Ainsworth sought to observe how the child responded to their mother by either seeking or resisting proximity, the ease with which they could be soothed and how quickly they returned to play. Ainsworth identified three kinds of attachment: Secure, Avoidant and Ambivalent Attachment.

Secure Attachment

This is found in children who have emotionally available, perceptive and responsive parents who are sensitive to their child's needs. In the Strange Situation, these children seek proximity, are soothed easily and quickly return to play.

This kind of secure foundation can allow children and the adults that they become, to feel safe and relaxed in the world. In relationships, people naturally seek closeness at times and separation at times, flowing easily between the two. They tend to feel safe and contained in expressing their emotions and carry a sense that their needs can be met in life. They also have a healthy exploratory drive allowing them to deeply explore areas of interest as well as to be adventurous and playful. People with secure attachment tend to have a healthy sense of self in which they can celebrate their strengths and acknowledge their limitations too.

Avoidant Attachment

This is a kind of insecure attachment found in children with parents who are emotionally unavailable, or who might reject, criticise or not respond to the child's emotional states. As a result there is a tendency in the child to withdraw emotionally, turning inwards to rely on him or her self to regulate emotional experience. This kind of parenting can value tasks over feelings, leading children to be more highly developed in their ability to function well in a practical way in the world and less developed in their ability to be aware of their emotions and to be empathic. In the Strange Situation, these children seemed to ignore the return of their parents and minimised proximity seeking.

Children with this attachment pattern can seem independent from early in life, but this autonomy is tied up with the wound of being left alone, at least with their emotional needs, earlier than they were ready for.

Ambivalent Attachment

This is a kind of insecure attachment found in children with parents who are inconsistently available, perceptive or responsive. It leads to a tendency in a child to protest or act out emotionally when loving attention is unpredictable. This protest aims to win back the attention of the parent. In the Strange Situation these children tended to be ambivalent towards proximity with their caregivers. They were also not easily soothed, as if they did not trust that the caregiver would stay long enough to soothe them sufficiently. Because of this, they did not readily return to play.

This kind of child tends to be emotionally sensitive, a quality originating in their need to monitor their caregiver and environment very closely to predict when love will go away. Because of this they learn to pick up on emotional cues, body language, sounds, sights or any slight nuances or changes in their environment. This can set off an internal alarm when love is no longer forthcoming, leading to crying, acting out or even hitting in order to attempt to restore connection and attention. Later in life this can evolve into a preoccupation with emotions in oneself and others and a tendency to interpret even the smallest cue as threatening. This kind of person can easily be distracted by emotions in and around them and prone to feeling emotionally overwhelmed.

Disorganised Attachment

A fourth kind of attachment called Disorganised or Disoriented Attachment was added later to Ainsworth's original work. It is also a form of insecure attachment occurring when there is so much fear or terror in the environment that there is not much for the baby to attach to. Even so, babies retain their primal need for connection and protection. So children can feel both comforted and frightened by their primary parent, who can act as both a figure of fear and reassurance for them. Their responses to caregivers can swing between Avoidant and Ambivalent styles of interaction with a conflicting mix of needs from a need to come close and a need to push or go away. This can cause great internal stress. These children can display a dazed look and sometimes seem either confused or apprehensive in the presence of a caregiver. Later in life this can cause so much fear and mistrust in relationships, rooted in their unresolved trauma, that it hinders their ability to connect and form enduring bonds with others.

Sometimes it is the environment that influences a Disorganised Attachment pattern, such as being born in the midst of war or when parents have unresolved trauma or take drugs, which can interfere with their ability to bond with their babies. Medical interventions that require repeated separation and handling of the baby by people other than their parents can also interfere with secure attachment and in some cases can trigger a Disorganised Attachment response. When a person experiences a traumatic event at any stage of life it can cause the nervous system and personality to disorganise, as happens with the Disorganised Attachment adaptation.

⇉ HOW THE NERVOUS SYSTEM AND BRAIN ARE SHAPED IN RELATIONSHIPS ⇇

With the field of neuroscience growing, Attachment styles can be explained on a physiological level. This gives us an empirical foundation for our emotional and relationship tendencies with each Attachment style priming the nervous system and shaping the brain and personality in a particular way.

SECURE ATTACHMENT
Secure Attachment leads to a healthy, balanced nervous system allowing us to feel safe and welcome in our world inside and out. We feel safe in expressing our emotions as well as in giving and receiving emotional support. A deep knowledge that relationships

can be nourishing, is carried with us. We have healthy access to all regions of our brains and to all levels of our experience including our feelings, instincts, thinking, and our ability to comfortably connect with others. This gives us emotional maturity for navigating life's ups and downs. It also can inspire us to live in line with our truth and values. Secure Attachment can be developed at any stage of life with the right kind of input.

All of us are human, with our hurts and challenges that have influenced our functioning. To create a bridge towards attaining Secure Attachment, Dr Stan Tatkin has come up with a reassuring term called Secure Functioning. It suggests that we all are able to function more securely no matter our history. This is as opposed to needing to aspire to some ideal state of Secure Attachment that might be elusive. So those of us whose brains have been wired towards Insecure Attachment (which to a greater or lesser extent is most of us) can be reassured that we can mature and our brains can rewire over time so that we feel that little bit more secure. We can do so by investing in the strategies offered in the next chapter, which work towards adding even a little more joy and connection to our lives.

Our Social Nervous System and Secure Attachment

The pioneering researcher, Dr Stephen Porges, shows us how very socially oriented our nervous systems are. His research investigated how a particular group of cranial nerves responds to our feeling safe or threatened. These nerves give us important information about our world and have a special sensitivity to our social world. They are the nerves that innervate our face and hands. When feeling safe and warmly connected with others, these nerves cause us to convey friendly facial cues, use a friendly, melodic tone of voice, and literally to hear each other better because our ears relax. Dr Porges has named this our Social Engagement System or Social Nervous System. When feeling threatened, the blood might feel like it drains from our face as we perhaps clench our jaw and tense up in preparation for fight, flight, freeze or faint survival responses. Dr Porges describes this as the nervous system devolving to more primitive functioning. At these times we lose contact with our Social Nervous System. So the key to accessing our Social Nervous System, is feeling safe.

Secure Attachment creates the conditions for developing a healthy Social Nervous System, also associated with optimal 'high' brain functioning. Fortunately it can be developed at any stage of life with the right kind of safe, caring input.

Even when our nervous systems are primed towards Insecure Attachment, we still have access to our Social Nervous Systems. This system is just not as well developed or as consistently available to us as with Secure Attachment.

When we can recognise what kinds of feelings the Social Nervous System generates, we can more easily learn to align with them. The more we do so, the more we can create neural connections that further develop our Social Nervous Systems, essentially rewiring our brains to function more optimally and resetting our experience of life to feel more harmonious and enriching.

How can we recognise our Social Nervous System? We can know it by that warm, fuzzy feeling when someone makes gentle eye contact with us and gives us a smile. It is the same kind of warm feeling that spreads through us when our feelings are acknowledged in a compassionate way, like when we are having a hard day and someone sees it and says, 'It's hard today, isn't it?' Pleasant feelings might rush through us. We might spontaneously take a deep breath of relief. The same heartfelt warmth can spread through us when someone takes our hand, just at the right time, for much-needed support, or when someone is willing to listen to our story. Pleasant, warm sensations spread through our face and body giving us a whole body experience of expanding, relaxing and slowing down. If we smile back, warmth and joy can expand even further. It is like an invisible relational field that flows between people when they are in rapport, invisibly knitting people together. It is the same way that a baby feels when they are seen, attuned to and lovingly treated by their caregiver. This is the Social Nervous System at work.

The purpose of the Social Nervous System is to promote social engagement for the sake of our survival as a species. In brainwave terms, we sink down into the slow waves of alpha, theta and perhaps delta too, bathing us in calm, creative and attuned presence. In this state many areas of the brain can be stimulated to work together in synchrony. In moments of complete absorption in rapport or creative flow, like in the midst of a rich conversation or while connecting with a loved one or when we are passionately and creatively absorbed in what we are doing, our slow brainwaves can spontaneously flip over into super-fast gamma brainwaves. This represents our capacity for super-thinking and compassion as well as opening us to inspiration, insight and a sense of flow. These spontaneous moments become more available to us and can be experienced more frequently when our Social Nervous Systems are well developed.

The more we orient ourselves towards the kinds of experiences that create these kinds of feelings, and spend time drawing on our warm memories too, the more we imprint these positive experiences in our brains, bodies and relationships. Dr Rick Hanson speaks of our brain's natural negativity bias. He believes we tend to focus on the negatives, like negative feedback, or that others are thinking negatively about us. At the same time we tend to marginalise the positives and forget the compliments and good feedback we might receive. Deliberately practising behaviours that feel warmly nourishing, such as spending quality time with important people in our lives, making a point of focusing on the positive things in our lives, practising random acts of kindness and recalling good, positive, warm memories when we are feeling down, can help us load up on the positives to counteract negativity. More ideas for boosting optimal Social Nervous System functioning, follow in the next chapter.

AVOIDANT ATTACHMENT

The parasympathetic nervous system is our calming nervous system. It gives us a healthy state of calm that can be stimulated in different ways. We can generate calmness in ourselves such as when we take a few deep breaths or spend time in nature. Our relationships can also help us to feel calmer and more emotionally contained as we support each other. With an Avoidant style, self-regulation of emotions and self-soothing become the default style for creating calm. This is as opposed to the possibility for co-regulation or supporting each other through emotional times. For a baby whose emotional needs are not sufficiently responded to, or responded to with criticism or negativity, self-regulation might have been the only option.

This learned style shapes the nervous system to quickly suppress emotional ups and downs with the result of keeping life at an even keel, stable and controlled. It can also shape a task-focused or intellectual individual because accomplishment of tasks can tend to be validated over emotions in this style of parenting. The task-oriented parts of the brain, associated with the left-brain hemisphere, develop to a greater extent than the emotion-oriented parts of the brain because they were relied upon more. This can also translate into being socially awkward to some extent and to being conflict averse so as to avoid emotional intensity. On the positive side this attachment adaption has gifts to give also. It can manifest as being really calm under pressure and remaining logical, organised, practical and task-focused in emotionally heated situations. The exception is when stress levels reach proportions too high even for this kind of person to cope, then primitive survival reactions such as a freeze response can take over.

In relationships it can translate into a tendency towards self-reliance and the individuals acting as if they have no need of others. This is in reaction to their thwarted attempts to reach out for care in their young, formative years. They learned instead to stop reaching out. It can also lead to a tendency to be dismissive of the emotional needs of others. Deep down, those with an Avoidant style do long for connection and do actively seek out a special person to be with. They just do not have an experience of relationships being nourishing, so they might settle into keeping their partner at some emotional distance and needing a fair amount of personal time and space. For the Avoidant type, a relationship ending through a break-up or divorce exposes the person's true yet previously hidden feelings of longing for a relationship. At these times an Avoidant person can even fall into a deep depression. Through healing experiences in relationships and practising behaviours that promote more secure functioning, this kind of person can learn to wake up into healthier, more connected relationship functioning, and rewire their nervous system and brain to function more effectively.

AMBIVALENT ATTACHMENT

The response of this attachment style to distress is to protest or act out as their sympathetic nervous system's fight or flight response is quickly activated. This is an attempt to restore the connection and attention that help them feel safe in the world. This was the baby's response to anxiety when their caregiver was inconsistent in meeting their needs. Because of this, a baby also learns that they cannot fully relax into trusting that their needs will be met consistently. In relationships later in life this can translate into a fear of abandonment, with a belief that the smallest removal of attention means abandonment or betrayal. Naturally this will make it more difficult for them to trust others and can also show up as clinginess or neediness. They know that relationships can be deeply nourishing, as they have experienced it. The challenge is that nourishment has become tied up with loss of it at unpredictable times.

The brain of the Ambivalent Attachment adaptation is seen to develop more in emotional regions, associated with the right brain hemisphere, than in task-focused areas. This is because the emotional level of experience was relied upon and responded to by their primary parent, or perhaps both of their parents, more so than their accomplishment of practical tasks. This can mean that a person is easily distracted when attempting to focus on tasks. Some common distractions are their own emotions or the emotions of others, as well as people, sounds and the environment around them.

Later in life this can manifest as preoccupation with emotions in oneself and others and an external focus (as opposed to the internal focus of the Avoidant style) for regulating emotions, such as needing others or circumstances to help them regulate their emotions. It causes a person to be emotionally sensitive and expressive with a tendency when emotions are heated to jump quickly to fight or flight. As adults this might turn into a tendency to shout or storm out of the room. This does not mean that this person should ignore their sensitive emotional radar. There are gifts in this too, such as being able to read people well and to be empathic. This can be fashioned into a valuable skill for facilitating insightful, empathic processes with individuals and between people, such as in couples or groups.

Through healing experiences in relationships and through practising behaviours such as offered in the next chapter, this kind of person can also learn to wake up into healthier, more trusting relationship functioning, rewiring their nervous system and brain to function in a more balanced way.

DISORGANISED ATTACHMENT

The nervous system of a person with this style of attachment becomes so conditioned to distress that they carry it around with them constantly, resulting in seeing danger in just about every little situation in their relationships and in the world. In other words their brains are just about constantly in a state of emotional flooding.

Through healing experiences in relationships, and perhaps with the help of psychotherapy that includes trauma resolution, it is also possible for this vulnerable and possibly highly resistant kind of person to wake up into healthier nervous system, brain and relationship functioning. What it takes is disentangling their natural pull towards attachment from their survival instincts. This can help them to internalise the difference between what is good for them and what is not good for them and what is truly (rather than imagined as) dangerous. With time this helps their nervous systems learn to regulate towards feeling calmer and more peaceful. This does take a lot of work around building safety into their minds, belief systems and bodies. But it is possible and can have rewarding effects on their quality of life and relationships.

LONG-TERM EFFECTS OF ATTACHMENT

An infant's attachment style is found to affect wellbeing and relationships throughout their life, in profound and enduring ways. It also can be passed on to future generations through the ability to promote secure attachment in one's own children.

Research suggests that a child's sense of security is as important to emotional and social wellbeing as actual safety is to physical wellbeing. Children assessed as Securely Attached at one year of age score higher on other measures later in childhood. These measures include self-esteem and having better social skills. Securely attached children are found to do better over time with being independent and resilient in the face of adversity as well as with emotional maturity and the ability to manage impulses and feelings. They are found to be more able to make and keep friendships, access empathy and compassion, make use of pro-social coping skills and maintain an optimistic outlook. They generally can find it easier to trust as well as to be intimate and affectionate. There is also a correlation between secure attachment and academic success.

With adolescents, Insecure Attachment is found to affect many areas including self-esteem, the ability to have long-term friendships, the emergence of chronic anxiety or depression, and it can also affect academic performance. With adults it is found that those with Secure Attachment as their base can recognise both the limitations and positive qualities of people in their lives as well as in themselves. They can be more forgiving of those around them and tend to value relationships more.

It is important to note that in the first few years of life an individual also forms attachment bonds with other caregivers or people they spend a lot of time with, such as their father, siblings and grandparents. These relationships may be different to the one with the primary caregiver and can lead a child to internalise more than one experience of what a relationship can be like. All of these relationships can influence future behaviour and social or relationship choices. Most of us do have a mix of different behavioural and emotional tendencies that can become active depending on our circumstances. For example, this can allow us to behave in a secure manner in some scenarios, anxious and fearful of abandonment in another scenario, and self-reliant and practical in yet another scenario.

Reflecting on merging and separation

Underpinning Attachment Theory is our relationship with life's cycles of merging and separation, or coming together and moving apart, which can be experienced in many aspects of life. Which feels more comfortable for you – merging or separation? How has this played out in your relationships intimately and professionally? Perhaps you tend to like closeness and when others don't feel the same it can feel unsettling. Or perhaps you like your space, feeling uncomfortable with too much human contact. Which is your preference?

ADULT RELATIONSHIP BLUEPRINT

Our original attachment style is found to influence our ability, throughout our lives, to be affectionate, feel understood, be comfortable with emotionality and intimacy, be able to talk about problems and concerns, and able to balance spending time apart with enjoying quality time together. Our adult relationships can also be a place for re-patterning our attachment styles to become more healthy and secure. Strategies for doing so follow in the next chapter.

There are many tools that have been created to assess the attachment style at play in adult relationships. An example of such a tool is a simple three-item questionnaire created in 1987 by researchers Cindy Hazan and Phil Shaver. They used it to investigate whether infant attachment style is still at work when, later in their lives as adults, they try to form intimate relationships. Their research found that some people do change their attachment style as they grow up, but the majority of adults choose the descriptor that matches the way that they were as children.

In adult romantic relationships the Secure Attachment style is characterised as generally friendly, trusting and happy. In these relationships, the people can see and accept that their partner is not perfect, perhaps with a view that their relationship is a place for both of them to learn and grow together through life experience and to support each other in living life to the full. Secure relationships tend to last longer than insecure relationships or at least to be more harmonious. According to Hazan and Shaver, those with a Secure Attachment style would find it relatively easy to get close to, and depend on, their partner. They are also comfortable with loved ones depending on them. Along with this they do not tend to worry about being abandoned or about feeling smothered when someone gets too close.

The Avoidant Attachment style is characterised by a fear of too much intimacy or closeness. These people tend to have a dismissive or fearful style towards emotions in themselves and others. They can live in a non-emotional way for stretches of time, although when they feel that their love is being threatened they can easily become jealous and anxious. Or when love is lost they can suddenly wake up to how much they wanted the person who has gone, which can lead to depression. Depression, or feeling lost, can lie deep beneath the surface of an Avoidant person because they have been disconnected from their feelings and from a belief that they need others. This can be shaped so early in life that they might not even be aware of why they feel this way and it can interfere with their ability to be emotionally available and intimate. According to Hazan and Shaver, those with an Avoidant Attachment style feel somewhat uncomfortable with closeness and can sometimes feel that others want more intimacy than they are comfortable with. They can also find it difficult to allow themselves to depend on others.

The Ambivalent Attachment style is characterised by anxiety and emotional preoccupation, which can interfere with trust and a sense of safety in the relationship.

These people can tend towards an obsessive view of love with a need for constant reassurance, reciprocation and validation. When this is not as forthcoming as they would like it to be, they can easily feel abandoned. Their emotions can swing regularly between emotional highs and lows, with elation when they feel validated, and despair when they feel abandoned. According to Hazan and Shaver, those with an Ambivalent Attachment style often worry about whether their partner really loves them and will stay with them. Their desire to merge or be in constant contact with their partner can sometimes scare people away.

REFLECTION

Do you see a pattern in the relationships you have attracted to date? What are recurring themes? Which attachment style or styles do you feel apply best to you and your loved ones?

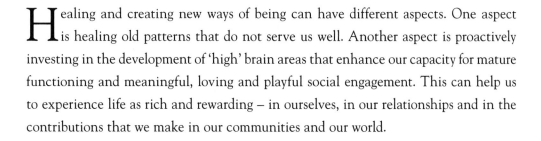

CHAPTER 8

Healing Old Patterns, Enhancing Vitality

*Healing is the process of re-establishing the integration
between body, mind and spirit, creating opportunities for the
return of the memory of wholeness.*

DAVID SIMON

H ealing and creating new ways of being can have different aspects. One aspect is healing old patterns that do not serve us well. Another aspect is proactively investing in the development of 'high' brain areas that enhance our capacity for mature functioning and meaningful, loving and playful social engagement. This can help us to experience life as rich and rewarding – in ourselves, in our relationships and in the contributions that we make in our communities and our world.

In support of both of these aspects, this chapter offers a range of options for you to pick and choose from. There are Mindful Body Moments that you can practise on your own and ones for practising in relationships. All of them offer proactive strategies for enriching and supporting your positive, vital experience of life. There are Mindful Body Processes, too, that you can try out to heal old emotional patterns and create new possibilities in your experience of life. There are also Mindful Body Reflections about some big challenges that many of us face, including depression and anxiety. The more we engage in these practices and reflections, the more old patterns will release their grip and be overlaid with positive impulses for connecting and responding.

⇛ SEVEN MINDFUL BODY MOMENTS ⇚

For incorporating into life

To follow are seven Mindful Body Moments intended as options for healing old patterns and opening to ever greater emotional and relationship nourishment. In the process we can rewire our brains towards optimal functioning and connecting. These Mindful Body Moments are not intended as a comprehensive list or to be followed in any particular order. As you read through the various options you are invited to consider which you might like to experiment with or apply in your life. As you move through your days you might also notice other opportunities, not included here, to invest in your vitality and emotional wellbeing. Therefore, treat these seven Mindful Body Moments as a guide to raising your awareness to the kinds of practices that support a healthy nervous system and brain. Feel free to add any meaningful moments that you come to yourself, to the list. An overview of the seven Mindful Body Moments included here are:

On your own

» 'Kind eyes'

» Noticing self-talk

» Making space for what you love

With each other

» Play!

» Marking transitions lovingly

» Making time to hear about each other's day

» Apologising and seeking repair soon

ON YOUR OWN

'Kind eyes'

One of the ingredients for Secure Attachment is a regular, loving gaze from mother or caregiver to baby. Attachment expert Dr Diane Poole Heller refers to this as a 'beam gleam' or an 'I'm special to you' gaze. If this was missing in your experience, it is possible to recreate it and feed it into your sense of self, now. Hopefully your current relationships offer moments of loving eye gaze that can help to repair old wounds. You can also use your imagination to help you here. To do so, imagine 'kind eyes' looking at you. This can be imagined as the loving gaze of a parent, or a friend who really loves you, or of a loving grandparent. Or you can picture the eyes of someone in your community who exudes kindness, or a spiritual leader who is truly compassionate and kind. For some, 'kind eyes' might be most easily imagined coming from a pet or an image of an animal. With the image of your choice, imagine that these 'kind eyes' are looking at you. Practise taking that gaze in, and softening into receiving its kindness. For others who are more auditory than visual, you can instead imagine hearing the voice of a loving, kind person speaking to you.

'Kind eyes' grows your ability to come from a softer, heart-felt space in relationships and life. Take a few moments to notice how your body responds to 'kind eyes'. You might notice your eyes feeling softer and that you gain a fuller, warmer sense of your body. You might feel your breathing become fuller too. There could also be a softening in your throat and belly as you take kindness in. Follow how your body responds for a few moments to really take in how you respond to this experience. Then see if you can look out into your day with even just a little more kindness in your eyes.

Next time you plan to speak with someone after an argument or perhaps when someone in your life is having a hard time, imagine 'kind eyes' before you go to them. Notice the effect on yourself and perhaps on the other person too, and notice how the conversation transpires. Sometimes without noticing it our body language, eyes and tone of voice can convey anxiety, tension or even subtle aggression. 'Kind eyes' can turn this around quickly and change how others experience us. Be kind to yourself in the process, too. It takes practice to sustain kindness. Even if you can achieve a few more seconds of coming from this kind place, it can make a big difference.

Noticing self-talk

Core beliefs can show up in the kinds of thoughts and conversations we carry in our minds. You may have come to believe you are good, wanted, worthy, competent and loveable, leading you to feel good in your body and your life, with a sense that relationships can be nourishing and that life is worth living. Or you may have come to believe that you are bad, unwanted, worthless, helpless or unlovable, leading you to feel uncomfortable in your body and unsettled in life, with a sense that relationships are problematic and life is hard and burdensome.

As you become skilled at catching your self-talk, you can practise turning an inner critic into an inner supporter. If you notice yourself thinking, I don't deserve this, or, I am ugly, notice how your body feels in response to these criticisms and then choose another thought that is positive, even if you cannot connect with it yet. Maybe you can frame the thought as a question to help you, such as, 'What if I am worthy?', or, 'What if I really am beautiful, especially to those who love me?' Then feel into how your body responds, and encourage these kinds of positive messages to stay with you for as long as you can. You might explore new possibilities such as being lovable, capable, or anything you like, and breathe your desired quality through you, to help you stand into it and become it more fully. You can also catch your body's reaction, first, and then notice the message relating to that reaction. So you might notice, 'Oh, I am standing like this and breathing like this and I feel tense or out of balance in this part of my body.' You can also notice the outlook that goes with the reaction and then choose a new way that you'd prefer to stand, look and breathe to seek an attitude adjustment.

Many times in this book you have been shown ways to change your body in order to change your mind, or to change your mind in order to change your body. Here is yet another reminder of your ability to do so, perhaps freeing even deep-seated beliefs, self-talk and postural habits to be more supportive and empowering.

Making space for what you love

Making time to explore and develop interests and talents can help us to feel inspired and fulfilled in a way that can spill over into our being warmly available for others. This also feeds a healthy sense of self. How much do you make time for the things you love? It could be family, a hobby or a form of creative expression, friends, your pets or spending time in nature. Or, for some, your work is your greatest love; perhaps you dream of making your passion your livelihood. There is no formula to tell you how much time you should spend doing the things you love. Perhaps make sure that each day factors in some quality time to invest in what brings you joy and fulfilment. This also extends to making time to give the people you love some quality attention regularly. Pausing for these kinds of Mindful Body Moments can feel like essential food for your heart and soul.

WITH EACH OTHER

Play!

Eye-to-eye, engaging, perhaps competitive, fun feeds our sense of loving, playful connection that can stimulate healthy brain- and nervous system functioning. Board games, sharing in sporting activities, getting on the floor with your children to join them in play, and even reading to each other, are many ways to have fun. The key is social engagement, as opposed to parallel play such as sitting in front of a computer screen or television together that does not encourage our interaction.

Marking transitions lovingly

Taking a few conscious moments to say hello and goodbye can be a meaningful way to acknowledge and support each other in the midst of life's comings and goings. This type of support grows a sense of loving connection and emotional support in your relationships. One idea is a 'Welcome Home Hug' as introduced by Stan Tatkin, relationship expert and author of *Wired For Love*. Tatkin speaks about how our nervous systems co-regulate when we exchange a belly-to-belly hug. He recommends it as a regular practice with our loved ones, such as on arriving home at the end of each day. The trick is to stay in the hug for long enough to feel your body soften and connect with your partner to get the full nervous system regulation effect. This can melt away tension while melting you both back into connection with each other and it only takes a few moments. You can also use this technique with your children by pausing to connect with them through a loving hug, held for long enough to sense your connection. For those not in an intimate relationship or without people to regularly connect with in this way, the touch chapter can help with this kind of nervous system regulation, by replacing hugs with the tangible support from your own hands.

Making time to hear about each other's day

Research has shown that if couples spend around 30 minutes talking with each other about their day, each day, it can contribute to a lasting and healthy relationship. This talking needs to be meaningful and touch on what has been on the other's mind and how they have felt through the day. Modern life places a lot of pressure on us. Making the time to connect is vital to sustain a sense of love and support. This applies to other important people in our lives, too, who we need to make regular time for – even if it's not daily. What does this have to do with the body? Making quality time helps to maintain our emotional attunement, our sense of connection and our loving supportiveness. It raises our oxytocin levels towards quieting the stress response and increases access to our mature prefrontal cortex and our Social Nervous System, supporting the development of both.

Apologising and seeking repair soon

Conflict is a natural part of living together. Disagreements will happen. The sooner we can find our way back to supporting each other, the sooner our negativity will leave and the better life will be for all parties. By being the 'bigger' person and apologising first, you can practise turning arguments around more quickly. Even if you believe it was not your fault, there usually is something you can own and apologise for. Maybe you weren't really listening or maybe you forgot to do something even if you had a valid reason, or maybe you said something hurtful even if you did not intend to. When one person apologises it can turn the whole energy in the room around, perhaps inviting the other person or people to do the same. This frees everyone's minds from emotional hijack, so that sensible solutions can be considered. Perhaps in the process we can all savour some heartfelt closeness. Not only does this feel good, investing in these moments also develops our Social Nervous System and hones our capacity for empathy and compassion. Any time we respond maturely it also develops our prefrontal cortex, which holds our most highly evolved capacity for brain functioning. Added to this, on a body level, releasing your stress response sooner is healthier for your body and mind. These are all good reasons to make the effort to be the 'bigger' person. The truth is, everyone makes mistakes and we can all learn and grow from our experiences.

⇉ FOUR MINDFUL BODY PROCESSES ⇇

To follow are four Mindful Body Processes that you can follow to heal old emotional patterns. It can feel overloading if you use all the processes at once. So choose the one that resonates with you most to try out first, and then perhaps try the others another time.

»   **Intervention of emotional memories:**
    This is a summary of a process offered earlier in the book in the emotions chapter, referred to as a 'Mindful Body Process towards emotional insight and transformation', with additional points added here.

»   **Visualisation for boosting self-esteem:**
    Explores boosting self-esteem, by calling to mind important people in your world.

»   **Internal support for those who really feel unsafe:**
    Provides a supportive internal strategy for people who may carry a lot of fear, anxiety and distress.

» **Cross-generational healing visualisation:**

An opportunity that all of us might benefit from – to ease family or generational tensions that have influenced us, whether we are aware of them or not. It is a gentle, loving process, which provides the image of ideal mothering to our entire lineage to bring us inner peace.

INTERVENTION OF EMOTIONAL MEMORIES

This is an effective way to work with your emotions and emotional tones, even if it's not clear where these emotions come from. This practice is supported in the science of neuroplasticity, which has revealed the brain to be receptive to change in the areas that store emotional memories and affect our emotional experience of life. This is provided we know how to engage with these stored memories. For a longer guided process, refer to the Mindful Body Process titled 'Towards emotional insight and transformation' in the chapter called 'Emotions and turning to the body'. To follow is a summary of this process as well as some additional points for clarification. The intention is to open us to the possibility of emotional healing and new, positive options for experiencing and responding in life.

Step 1: Identify a familiar feeling

Identify an emotion that you wish to understand more deeply and perhaps change. You might choose depression, emotional numbness, anxiety, panic, anger, irritation, or any other feeling you carry with you and are curious to explore. Then pause to allow the feelings to grow in your body and mind so that you can really feel them.

Step 2: Consider the original trigger

Consider the triggers for your feeling this way, scanning back in time through your memories of times you felt this way. Consider where this feeling originated, as if you could find an original trigger for feeling this way. Or you could consider what your earliest memory is of feeling this way. This might bring just a sense (not necessarily a clear memory) of an earlier time in life when you felt this way. Be open and spontaneous with what comes to mind. It might be an actual event or it might simply be a sense of a time in your life. Perhaps it was before you were five years old or before you were ten years old, or maybe later in life. No matter how much information you recall, spend some time letting a picture develop in your mind. Piece together as much information as you can about where you were, what was happening, who was there and what part of the experience you noticed most strongly. If your memory is not clear, and to help you make implicit, non-verbal or felt memory into explicit, verbal memory so that it can be acknowledged and integrated into your 'high' brain's awareness, it can be helpful to create a statement that represents your experience and what it has meant for you. Examples might be: 'I am all alone with nobody to help me, so I must be worthless', or, 'When I say or do something freely it makes people angry and they leave, so I would rather be passive', or, 'I am so mad that it happened to me. Life is so unfair.' This statement is an attempt to make the unconscious conscious. It does not need to make perfect sense; it just needs to feel like a good fit for your emotional experience and the conclusions about people or life that you might have come to. You might realise how these feelings and beliefs have influenced your life, at least some of the time.

Step 3: Insert resources into your memory using your imagination

It is time now to intervene imaginatively to positively affect the outcome of this memory that has probably influenced your emotional tone and your life in some way. To do so you might imagine a supportive or protective figure appearing. This figure might finally be able to fight for what's fair, or help you when you feel passive, or nurture you towards feeling worthy. Let whoever or whatever arrives be a perfect remedy for your needs, now, which is something you might take a few moments to imagine and feel into. Then notice what happens for you when this figure is with you, inserted right into the memory you are working with. How does your body respond and how does it feel for the younger version of yourself to receive this in the context of your memory? What effect does it start to have on the experience? For maximum impact it is important to pause to feel into your body now and again, perhaps using breathing, posture and some movement to help you do so. This step begins a process necessary for brain change, which is to begin to juxtapose new, positive experience with old experience. In this case you are applying a specific remedy, using imagination to meet the emotional needs of a specific time in your past. This juxtaposing new with old will continue in Step 4, and allows for new neural pathways to replace old ones so that when you recall the memory you will start to recall the intervention, too. Doing so can start to ease and release old beliefs, old ways of reacting to life and age-old emotional tendencies.

Step 4: Imagine victory and feeling safe

Follow through with your imagination to the point where, related to your original memory, you feel victorious and safe and eventually perhaps even at peace, or happy. Allow the scene to unfold in your imagination as if you were watching a movie in which you are a central actor and in which you go slowly enough to really feel into the shifts in the scenario. Allow yourself to be supported or defended, your situation to be overcome and a triggering person or people to be well taken care of in whatever way feels good. Let your imagination, with the help of your supportive or protective figure, guide you towards overcoming your challenges, one step at a time. When you have reached a place that feels positive and strong, you are ready to close your exploration. To do so, you are invited to find a posture or hand gesture that represents how the final positive outcome feels. This will become a Mindful Body Moment for you to recall in Step 5.

Step 5: Remind yourself of the positive posture or gesture in the days that follow

Make use of your representative posture or gesture as a Mindful Body Moment for at least 30 seconds, whenever you think of it or in support of when you might feel emotional in a similar way in future. You might also wish to write a note to yourself or find a picture or a quote that represents your new positive, and place it where you can see it regularly. These can all be reminders of your new positive state.

Step 6: Evaluate your progress over time

The impact of your emotional transformation might drift out of your awareness in the weeks that follow. You may find that you forget to use your Mindful Body Moments, too, which is natural. You can, however, still notice long-lasting shifts. You might wish to make a note in your diary to reflect, perhaps a month from now, on how your experience and response to life might have been influenced. This allows you to evaluate the effectiveness of the process and might also encourage you to repeat the process if you feel there is more work to be done. Repeating the process can also reinforce or strengthen the positive emotional outcome in relation to certain feelings that you might know well.

If at any stage you experience resistance to this process, consider starting from step one again, using your resistance as the emotional tone to explore. This honors that resistance can be a valid experience at times in our lives too, with a story to tell about your life, such as about a time when situations felt too painful to bear. Resistance can protect us like an emotional shield, helping us live through challenging times. There also might come a time when this shield is no longer necessary for our circumstances and can hold us back from living life to the full.

VISUALISATION FOR BOOSTING SELF-ESTEEM

Who are the people you carry with you in your mind? Take a few moments to scan your mind for who might be with you today. As part of how we are wired for connection, we gather in our minds a community of people who have made an impression on us. This allows us to call them to mind at will and feel as if they are with us. It is how a baby comes to remember that their mother still exists when she is not in the room, and it is how we learn to tell friend from foe. This ability is a function of mirror neurons that allow our brains and bodies to record images of key people in our lives. These mental photographs capture how they look, feel and sound to us. As we move through life our internal community grows. In this way we are always accompanied by the imagined presence of many people.

For some, however, the influence is not always positive. Many of us have had negative experiences that we have also internalised. Perhaps these experiences started early in life and were based on other people's reactions to us. These memories can turn into a loud inner critic, or old, familiar and upsetting feelings visiting us regularly and making us feel awful. Luckily we have it in us to sway our internal community towards the positive, by consciously bringing to mind people who make us feel good about ourselves. They are the people, real or imagined, who truly love us, value us and make us feel safe. We can also add loved pets or spiritual figures, or anyone or anything that feels supportive. Filling our minds with these positive influences can be a buffer against negativity, from the inside out. They can help us to feel supported even when we are on our own, and these influences can boost our self-confidence and self-worth when we need a lift.

The visualisation

Take a few moments to recall people in your life who absolutely warm your heart. They might include family or extended family members, or someone in your community who has helped you and valued you. It might be a teacher who really saw and understood you, or a special friend or friends. It could even be a movie character who inspires you, or a spiritual figure. You could also recall a loved pet. For some, being in nature warms their hearts. It does not matter what you imagine or how many images you carry inside (some carry just one wonderful image of one person or being or place; others like to populate their inner world with many happy things). The only thing that matters is that the thought of it warms your heart and makes you feel special, safe and deeply accepted for who you are.

Notice what happens in your body and mind as you allow this influence to sink in. Let the feelings spread through you to fill more of your body and being. Soak it all up and notice how and where it settles in your body. What does this picture give you? Perhaps it gives you some inner peace or warm joy, perhaps relief and more hope. Feel into what is true for you. Remember to hold this image and the body experience of it for at least 30 seconds to really allow it to register in your body and brain.

You are welcome to use this visualisation as often as you like, especially if your inner community has been populated by negative, critical voices. This can help you make a habit of connecting with your feel-good inner community. If you are going through a difficult time you could integrate this visualisation as a short practice each day, such as into your morning routine to set a warm tone for the day. Maybe you could also place photographs of special people or things where you can see them regularly at home and work and consciously pause now and again to take in their warmth. Doing these kinds of things can strengthen your loving sense of self, boost your self-esteem and offer a mental sounding board when you need one, such as asking 'What would you do?', or 'What do you suggest I do?', when you need guidance.

Case study 9: Linda's story

After Linda's mother had passed away two years before, Linda found a way to reconnect with her mother on an emotional level. Since her mother died, Linda had been on a gradual decline in her ability to cope emotionally, and especially in her stressful job. She was a fighter and her fight was being triggered regularly by all the pressure at work and the anxiety of potential redundancies. She felt under constant pressure to add value at work or risk losing her job. She used to have a person in her office that she could talk to openly, and laugh with about their situation, for some relief. But that person no longer worked there. Linda's mother used to be that person for Linda, too. She could make Linda laugh at herself and her situation and offered a perspective of life that was always relieving. Linda used to speak to her mum every day. When her mum passed away she lost an enormous part of her world, including her sense of stability and her ability to cope with stress. She dreamed of leaving her stressful job, but she felt too dependent on it because it provided for her family. She just wished she had someone in her office she could talk to and laugh with, to ease the pressure. She spoke of feeling in a state of panic a lot of the time. When we spoke about what her mum might have suggested she do, she immediately softened. She gave herself some advice from her mother's perspective that resonated with her. She said that her mum always knew what to say. One of the ideas that came from this discussion was to keep a picture of her mum on her desk, as a reminder of this enormously supportive person. It was like a light went on inside Linda when she realised that she could still carry her mother with her. She knew one day she wanted to leave her job to find a more positive environment to work in, but for now, imagining her mum was with her was all she needed. Advice her mum might give her would be to seek out people at work she could talk to and be supported by. She hoped to find this one day, but in the meantime the urgency for support was quieted simply by the feeling of her mother's presence.

INTERNAL SUPPORT FOR THOSE WHO FEEL REALLY UNSAFE

This process again refers to how, throughout our lives, we internalise and accumulate a community of people who have made an impression on us. In this process the focus is on supporting those who might have had a lot of negative influence or trauma. For people who might have this experience, feeling safe is a big and important aspiration. In these cases, transforming an internal community that includes terrifying mental intrusions might require professional support. One helpful practice that can complement professional guidance is to imagine inserting a strong protective figure into your mind's internal community, to stand between you and what you fear. You could choose any image that works for you. It could be a person who you feel really cares about you and has your best interests at heart, or a spiritual figure, or even a wild animal. Some find the image of a tiger helpful, with its confident stride and regal beauty representing boldness and the ability to be fierce too, in this case in service of self-protection. Use whatever works for you. Remember to take a few moments to let the feeling of its presence seep into your body and being. If you wish, you can imagine a positive scenario unfolding as your protector helps you come out victorious in relation to your fears.

It is important to reiterate that this mental buffer against negativity is not meant to replace taking the steps to find professional or social support to resolve your fears more fully. It is meant as a quick way for you to perhaps boost courage and confidence so that you no longer feel immobilised by your fears. Practising this visualisation and anchoring it in your mindful body, can also be a visceral reminder that protection is possible. The world can start to feel even a tiny bit safer.

CROSS-GENERATIONAL HEALING VISUALISATION

You cannot give what you did not get. Parents most of the time are doing the best that they can in their circumstances. Parents have their own set of parents who in turn have their own background and life experience to contend with. So can you blame your parents for all of your emotional wounds? The answer is no. When you find out their story and history it can awaken your compassion for them and their history, which can extend further back in generations than is possible to remember. Acknowledging your background is a first step towards healing, so that you know what you are working with. Then it is up to you to take responsibility for your experience of life and your behaviour. In this you strive towards the change that will make your life, and the life of the generations that follow you, richer and more enjoyable.

Because so many of us come from ancestry where there has been suffering, whether in our immediate family or in generations before, the following visualisation can offer welcome relief. It is designed to provide a sense of support and wholeness as we integrate ourselves into the generations of family that came before us. Even if parents struggled with their ability to love their children, imagining them with their parents behind them and their parent's parents behind them, and so on, all standing behind each other, can reconstitute our ancestry in a stable way that has strength in numbers. This can help to build a new mental picture and body sense of support into our experience of our history. It can also build in us a sense of innate belonging, no matter how we were treated by our parents. We can come to realise that it is our turn, now, to influence our own lives and the generations that follow us. It is our turn to make our mark.

Visualisation

Find a comfortable sitting position and bring attention to your breathing for a few moments. Then notice your heart. Imagine breathing for a few moments through your heart, giving space to all the feelings you find there.

Now imagine you are standing, facing forwards, looking out over a beautiful horizon. With your imagination, bring your parents in to stand behind you. If you had more than one set of parents place them all behind you. They don't need to say anything or be any way, simply feel their presence standing behind you, also looking forwards out over the horizon. Then add their parents behind them, so that you have your parents behind you and your grandparents behind them. Let them all gaze forwards out over the horizon in a pyramid of people expanding out behind you. Now slowly imagine the parents of your grandparents standing behind them. Picture it in your mind in your own way – you might not know what they looked like, but that's OK. Continue growing your family, including their parents standing behind them and so on, for endless generations, to form a pyramid shape expanding out behind you of which you are the point. Let the pyramid grow wider and wider and spread further and further back until it dissolves into the furthest horizon behind you.

Feel the presence of this very large group of people. Allow them all to be who they are and who they were with all that they may have gone through and all that they may have done. Feel the strength of having such a large group behind you. You are a product of this ancestry. You belong. And you are the one in the front, now, leading your way.

Now imagine a mother figure, one who is big, warm and unconditionally loving. Let this wonderful mother take shape from the horizon behind all of you. She grows to surround and embrace you all. She holds with big, loving arms, a warm, welcoming body and compassionate, pervasive presence. Her energy permeates all of you to glow through all of your hearts. Grow this image for a few moments, soaking up the feeling of it. Breathe it in and breathe it out. Breathe in love. Breathe out love. Breathe in peace. Breathe out peace. Feel full of heart and warmth.

Finally, imagine a protective, heavenly father energy surrounding the loving, embracing mother image. Let this protective masculine energy provide strength and balance to the feminine hold. This synergy represents the ultimate supportive union of masculine and feminine, as if they are heavenly parents to hold you and your ancestry. Be with this image for a few more moments with the presence of both a mother and a father in archetypal perfection, whatever that looks like for you.

Then, when you feel ready, notice your body. How do you feel and where in your body can you sense these feelings? Place your hand or both hands on any area of your body that feels comfortable. Perhaps ask for an image that can fit in your heart to help you remember this experience and carry it with you. When you are ready, stretch out your body and take a few deep breaths before moving out into your day or night.

This visualisation can be done just once, potentially with a long-lasting effect, or you are welcome to repeat it as many times as you wish, to feel supported, held and empowered in this intergenerational way.

⟫ TWO MINDFUL BODY REFLECTIONS ⟪

The following Mindful Body Reflections are opportunities for insight through reflection on various topics. Rather than offering specific advice, reading them is intended to stimulate your thinking and speak to ideas that could be helpful from a mindful body perspective.

» Seeing through depression and anxiety: Reflections on depression and anxiety and the roots of these conditions in attachment styles.

» A story about different relationship styles and what is needed for change: Reflections on one way that Insecure Attachment styles can interact in relationships, pointing to what is needed for lasting change.

SEEING THROUGH DEPRESSION AND ANXIETY

Depression and anxiety are so prevalent throughout the world nowadays that it probably says more about the way of the world than about our upbringing. This might be because we live in a world that is becoming more and more detached from nature, both in terms of the natural world and in terms of what is natural for us as humans. Our modern lives can place unnatural pressure on us to the point that we can fall prey to anxiety and depression as symptoms of chronic stress. All of our rushing around and being so busy can take away valuable time for rest, integration, play and recuperation.

Anxiety is a stress response involving low-grade, sometimes chronic activation of the sympathetic nervous system. This keeps stress hormones like cortisol flowing through our bodies and affects our brains with some degree of emotional flooding. This limits our access to 'high' brain reasoning and insight. When more highly activated, such as in panic, the sympathetic nervous system moves into fight or flight mode. Anxiety is more of a lingering condition than the fleeting urgency of panic. With anxiety we can feel as immobilised as when we are depressed. Depression involves chronic over-activation of the parasympathetic nervous system that can lead to lethargy and that also limits access to our 'high' brains because of some degree of emotional flooding.

These two styles of nervous system over-activation resemble the Insecure Attachment styles of Ambivalent (tending towards anxiety) and Avoidant (tending towards depression). Perhaps a foundation is set in our formative years predisposing us to anxiety or depression later in life. It is also the case that at any stage of life anxiety can be triggered. All it takes, which is similar to the Ambivalent style of attachment, is regularly inconsistent and unpredictable input. Think traffic jams, workplace redundancies, illness, or tension flair ups at home or work. Depression can also be triggered at any stage of life when life feels regularly cold or emotionally neglectful, which is similar to the Avoidant Attachment style. This can happen when people are so busy and stretched, and more inclined to text or tweet than to meet in person, or when financial pressures lead us to lose touch with ourselves, including our passions and sense of meaningful purpose.

These are some of the big issues facing humanity. When our nervous systems are more balanced it helps us face life's challenges more skillfully. We have good access to our 'high brains', we are better able to navigate life's ups and downs and to return to a state of calm more quickly after being triggered. Whether it is our original Secure Attachment style that helped us achieve this or our personal growth later in life, this is key to our ability to respond to daily stressors in resourceful ways.

With both anxiety and depression, turning to the body, away from the stories of the mind, can be half the battle won. This is because, on a body level, there is always something you can do to change how you feel. Sometimes support is needed when what is inside feels too big and scary to confront alone. Professional support and perhaps medication are valuable resources at these times. Then, as you find your ability to look inwards, touch and transform what you find inside, and anchor your attention in your grounded, present body, it can feel like coming back to life. From there your mindful body can become your trusted friend on a meaningful journey through life.

Upbringing is not the only factor that can predispose us to depression, anxiety or secure emotional resilience; there are themes from Attachment Theory that can still be helpful to consider. The questions that follow reflect these themes. Together with the body-based reflections they can prove helpful in times of anxiety or depression.

Anxiety

Some questions based on the Ambivalent Attachment style that could be helpful are: 'What is it I fear will be taken away?', or, 'What is it that is changing, now, that feels threatening?' and perhaps, 'What is the worst that could happen?' (as asked in the stress chapter related to anticipatory stress). As a child you might have felt helpless to do anything about situations. You might consider, 'If my mature self could give my more vulnerable or immature self some advice, what would it say?'

On a body level, action can negate anxiety. Action gets you out of your thoughts and mobilises you to at least begin to do what you need to. Even completing daily chores or getting through your to-do list can have a relieving effect on anxiety. Getting into action activates the sympathetic nervous system more fully so that your fighting spirit is mobilised and your body can then discharge sympathetic nervous system activation. With action you signal to your brain that you are not helpless, that you can take strides towards taking care of yourself. In the process, you can get a dopamine 'I did it!' feeling to motivate you to continue taking proactive steps to achieve goals and resolve challenges. Once you have gained a few wins, you can grow more confident in your ability to navigate anxiety and so become more emotionally resilient.

To combat chronic anxiety, embark on some physical exercise that focuses on strength and awareness in your lower body. Running and Tai Chi are two examples, or you can simply emphasise your legs while exercising in your preferred way. Anxiety tends to constellate in your upper body, so focusing on your legs can help ground the rising energy of anxiety. This can have an energising and motivating effect.

Depression

In keeping with themes of the Avoidant Attachment style, at the root of depression can lie feelings of isolation and helplessness, tied up with an inability to reach out for support. Consider, 'Am I really helpless now?' and 'Who are the people or places that I might be able to turn to for support?' This could take different forms, such as people in one's life, a spiritual community, participating in hobbies, or psychotherapy – whatever feels right for you. It can be no small task for some people to do this. Take baby steps in ways that feel safe, to let some light into your bubble of isolation. Hopefully these small steps can motivate you to continue. In the process, you can begin to wake up to your feelings and tune in to your values, dreams and creative spirit again.

On a body level, getting moving in any way helps to clear out the cobwebs of a depressed body-mind. It is well-known that regular physical exercise can combat depression. Any action activates the sympathetic nervous system. This can counter the tendency towards lethargy from over-activation of the parasympathetic nervous system. Exercise also tops up our feel-good hormones. As we start to feel safer and more motivated to come out of isolation, we can also feel more empowered to make changes that we might long for. This can be satisfying, uplifting and motivating. It can feel like we've created ourselves anew.

⇒ A STORY ABOUT DIFFERENT RELATIONSHIP STYLES ⇐

WHAT IS NEEDED FOR CHANGE

(adapted from a story by Dr Harville Hendrix)

A Turtle and a Hailstorm fall in love. When things are good, all is happy. When they fight, that is when problems arise because their styles of conflict are different. Turtle generally withdraws into its shell and Hailstorm generally hails down in fury. Over time, all it took was a hint of withdrawal or hail to spark conflict. Over time, this led to more frequent discord in their relationship. Each wished that the other would change, as if that would solve all of their problems. But nothing changed until a wizard appeared and helped them understand how things could be different. The wizard explained that each had a valid reason for behaving as they did, based on how they had learned to survive in life. What was needed was for both to develop new skills for being with each other when feelings got heated. For Turtle this meant having the courage to stay out of its shell to maintain connection with Hailstorm. This could allow Hailstorm to feel met and reassured. For Hailstorm it meant learning to contain its hail from doing damage. In so doing it could help Turtle feel safer to stay in contact. This meant that both could grow towards overcoming their old survival patterns, have less conflict, and build a greater sense of closeness in their relationship. It also meant that both could be more fulfilled in their individual lives as each explored living into their fuller potential. For Turtle this might mean growing more assertive, sociable and comfortable with intimacy and for Hailstorm it might mean feeling more emotionally contained and supported towards feeling more trusting and relaxed in life.

Reflection

We are in relationships in different ways in our lives – as couples, children, siblings, parents, friends, co-workers and more. With attention we can come to notice how we have patterns of behaviour that recur in our relationships. Even though we can behave differently at times, most of us do tend towards a dominant style. This short story told by Dr Harville Hendrix, creator of Imago Relationship Therapy, speaks to two Insecure Attachment styles, an Avoidant Turtle and an Ambivalent Hailstorm, as two common styles in relationships and how they can play out in conflict.

As you read the story you might have identified with one or the other as representing your tendencies in relationships. Or you might be able to recognise a little of each character in your different relationships. Or if you are young and have not had much experience in intimate relationships, you might recognise a family pattern of reaction and find yourself somewhere in that, too. Or you might notice how you tend to be with friends. Which one describes you best?

The story also points out that the key to lasting change is mutual support and cooperation. How might you apply some of this wisdom in your relationships? Is there something, even something small, that you can try to do differently? Take a risk and be curious about the effect.

On a body level it makes good sense to move towards mutual growth and support. Our nervous systems are directly affected by the nature of our relationships and can either support and contain us, or agitate and upset us. It is not about passing moments but rather about what our relationships are like most of the time. Are we regularly feeling emotionally flooded? Or is our normal a calm, connected space? Ultimately, seeking greater harmony in our relationships and sometimes making hard choices about staying with, or leaving, the relationships we are in, can be what changes the quality of our lives. If we can feel more supported in our relationships, this can be a catalyst for improving physical and emotional health and promoting the clear functioning of our minds.

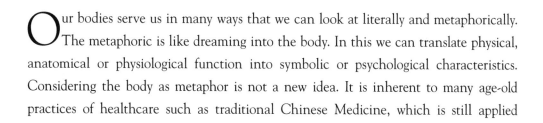

CHAPTER 9

Ailments and Injuries as Metaphors for Life

Uncover the wisdom in your wounds, the blessings in your misfortunes, and the gifts that are waiting to be claimed where you may least expect them, in the dark. If shadows could talk, they would tell you that there is gold to be mined in every experience.

DEBBIE FORD

Our bodies serve us in many ways that we can look at literally and metaphorically. The metaphoric is like dreaming into the body. In this we can translate physical, anatomical or physiological function into symbolic or psychological characteristics. Considering the body as metaphor is not a new idea. It is inherent to many age-old practices of healthcare such as traditional Chinese Medicine, which is still applied today as it was centuries ago. According to Dianne Connelly, author of *Traditional Acupuncture: The Law of the Five Elements*, 'The skin is not separate from the emotions, or the emotions separate from the back, or the back separate from the kidneys, or the kidneys separate from will and ambition, or will and ambition separate from the spleen, or the spleen separate from sexual confidence.' From this perspective, body, mind, emotions and spirit are seen as different expressions of the same thing. Another age-old example is the approach of Hippocrates, the father of Western medicine, who lived centuries ago. He held a holistic and systemic view of healthcare. Many factors were considered in the care of patients – many factors contribute to a particular ailment. A patient might be asked about their temperament or their living conditions, the weather patterns at the time or the social or political circumstances that might play a part in a person's malaise.

⇾ BODY AS METAPHOR ⇽

In the seventeenth century the philosopher, Rene Descartes, popularised a dualistic view of mind and body, as separate. This led to centuries of advances in the field of medicine that have improved quality of life and healthcare. Descartes' theories have also led to developments in the field of psychology.

Over the last half-century or so, these holistic approaches have made a comeback and are readily applied to understanding how the mind and emotions influence physical health. Early research started with the correlation of stress with symptoms like high blood pressure, heart disease and the Type A personality. There was also the discovery many years ago of the placebo effect, where simply a belief that medicine is received can at times lead to recovery. More recently, a holistic perspective is gaining credibility through fields like psychoneuroimmunology, which provides a scientific basis for how emotions affect health and physiological functioning. The result is a more widely recognised shift from viewing the body mechanistically. The body is no longer something to maintain and fix. It is now viewed more subjectively and soulfully as *somebody* – you. Many practitioners are opening to the possibility that symptoms are biofeedback letting us know how life is affecting us at the time. In this way our bodies are seen as dynamic, living expressions of us.

Understandably, every field of study requires experts, so consulting with medical professionals for their valuable contribution is important. Each profession has an important part to play. At the same time you can also find your own way of viewing your body symptoms as meaningful. In this you can reflect on the possible life metaphor associated with your symptoms, asking questions like 'Why this part of my body?' and 'Why now?' This way you are engaging with your symptoms and using them to inspire personal change in support of your recovery or quality of life. This can help to speed up recovery. Or it can simply help you be more optimistic, as you find comfort in the belief that what you are going through is happening for a reason, even if you cannot see it fully yet.

DID YOU CAUSE YOUR SYMPTOMS?

The idea that you caused your symptoms, is controversial, especially when it comes to children who are ill or when bad things happen to good people. A more useful view is that symptoms can happen for reasons beyond what we might ever know. So our task is to consider how to respond to what happens, in constructive, helpful ways.

Symptoms may be influenced by our state of mind at the time, such as when we stub a toe or trip while lost in thought. Immunity is also seen to be affected by our state of mind and emotions. For example, research suggests we are more prone to the common cold when there has been fighting in the home or when we have been feeling down. Symptoms can also be connected with relationships, so a pain in our necks, on closer inspection, might link to worry about a child or to feeling guilty about something. From a Family Constellations perspective, physical illness and emotional tendencies can be passed down from generation to generation, so that symptoms might carry stories from very long ago that can affect our lives now. As part of a holistic approach to treatment, Family Constellations hones in on possible family and trans-generational influences that could play a part in the formation of symptoms and illness. Examples of such influences are trauma associated with a family losing a loved one, or war that has left enduring scars on a family and that can influence health. In traditional medicine, genes of course play a significant role, too, in specific illnesses.

Searching for an original cause of our symptoms is tricky and perhaps we will never know what caused our sickness. The only thing that is important is finding meaning and relief through whatever approach works for us.

⇒ MINDFUL BODY PROCESS ⇐

How to make ailments and injuries meaningful

Your ailments and injuries urgently pull your attention into your body. First, if need be, seek appropriate help, medical or otherwise. Then, when the time is right, your symptoms may offer an opportunity for self-reflection that can yield interesting results. What in your life might be mirrored by the aches and pains? Why now? How can you be with your body and your situation supportively?

You might discover the need for change in the way that you are going about this moment (for example if you stub your toe you might be invited to slow down). Or you might discover a need to change the way you are going about your week (for example if the flu is forcing you to take it easier). Or body tension and aches might invite you to do some gentle stretching or exercise. If your situation is severe, calling for deep soul searching towards changing your priorities or the way that you live your life may be necessary. Sometimes you can only see in retrospect how accidents or illnesses open you to untapped potential or to a new path and quality of life that you would not have discovered otherwise. This belief, that things happen for a reason, takes faith and a positive outlook that can assist healing. This is as opposed to negativity and despair, which are found to weaken your immune response, slow down the rate of your recovery or detract from the quality of your life.

You may not always be able to 'cure' your ailment or fully repair your injury, but you can always work with your attitude and choose to look for opportunities and life lessons. To help you extract meaning from symptoms and perhaps find a life lesson, here is a set of questions that can guide you:

1) WHAT IS YOUR SYMPTOM? DESCRIBE YOUR SENSATIONS

This could be anything from tension, discomfort and tiredness, to aches, pains, injury or illness. Use descriptive words, images or sounds to identify your bodily sensations and notice how your posture might be affected. For example, you might feel 'tense in your shoulders and like you're holding so much together' or 'throbbing as if a hammer is hitting your head' or 'sensitive and wobbly so you can't walk properly' or 'heavy and weighed down', or you could apply simple, descriptive words like pressure, tingling, stabbing, aching or whatever feels right.

2) WHAT PART OF YOUR BODY IS AFFECTED AND WHAT MIGHT THE METAPHOR BE?

How might your descriptive words and the literal function of the affected area apply to your life? With this enquiry you can explore playing with words and ideas until something resonates. If your eye is affected, its function is sight or vision. So if you have injured your eye, you might consider what you are not willing to see, right now in your life? Or is there something that you are afraid for others to see about you? Perhaps the metaphor 'eyes as a window to your soul' is applicable. If you have a headache, your brain is housed there, or your intelligence and your thinking. So if you have a headache that feels like a clamp applying pressure to your head, you might consider how your thinking might be putting pressure on you. What area of your life might this apply to? A splitting headache could reflect something about feeling divided or ambivalent in some area of your life. Remember it is not about getting it 'right'; it is more about associating personal relevance to why this might be happening to you now. If it is an internal organ, the same applies. For example, your lungs are involved in breathing as well as the metaphors of inspiration and letting go. Your digestion processes what you ingest or take in from the outside, and your heart pulses lifeblood through your body and also plays a role in responding to your feelings. If you don't know the function of an organ in your body, you can simply think about the area where it is located in general terms, and how you associate with the area. For example, the gut could reflect your gut feelings. Or you can simply consider how your descriptive words might apply to your life; how might the words 'sharp stabbing pain' apply to your life? Or how might the words 'dull chronic ache' be reflected in an area of your life? You will still be able to extract relevance and then you can simply move on to the next question, where you come up with a constructive response or action plan.

COMMON BODY METAPHORS

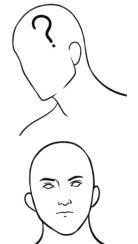

The following are some common metaphors associated with different body parts. This is not meant as a comprehensive list. Rather, the intention is to spark your imagination and curiosity about your body as a reflection of an aspect of your life.

Head

Thinking. What is the nature of your self-talk lately? Our heads can also reflect our relationship with spirituality or our higher self.

Face

Expressing, sensing (hearing, seeing, tasting, smelling) and communicating

Neck

Head–heart connection and throat as communication

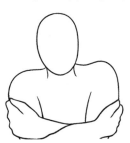

Shoulders

How we shoulder burdens and responsibilities and how what we do is aligned with our hearts. Your upper arms and shoulders are closer to your heart, which could reflect whether your heart is invested in what you are doing. Are you giving and receiving in harmony with your heart? Or are you feeling guarded, unsafe, or unsure in some way that limits your desire to reach out?

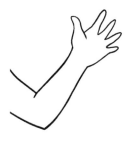

Arms and hands

Doing and relating, giving and receiving in relationships and work. Your fingers and hands actually touch people and your world and so could reflect your attitudes about the details of what you are working on and your feelings about giving and receiving. Your elbows can also tell stories relating to personal space or 'elbow room'.

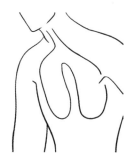

Upper torso

Lungs can relate to your relationship with life's cycles of inspiration and letting go. Which end is more challenging for you? Breathing also opens you to feeling your emotions, or restricts and limits your emotional experience. How might this be meaningful for you? Heart relates to all matters of emotion and love. The front of the chest is where your heart faces the world, possibly relating to how you face the world and show your heart. The back of the chest can be where you store past hurts as tension. Your solar plexus area holds a bundle of nerves that can be a target for anxiety. This area can also reflect your relationship with your instincts or gut feelings, which you can be open to or shut off from. It is the area that sits between your heart's feelings and your gut instincts. This area can either feel connected and in harmony or closed and conflicted.

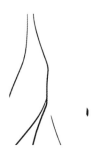

Lower torso

Many organs live here including your digestive organs. It is where a lot of your emotional experience gets processed. This brings to mind queries about how you are digesting or 'stomaching' your experience or generally processing different emotions. Core strength resides here and the area just under your navel is also considered in some traditions to be your body's vital energy centre. How you are feeling in this area can reflect your relationship with personal power and self-containment.

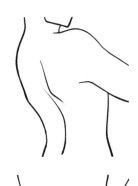

Spine

Support. What is your relationship with being and feeling supported? What is your relationship with feeling able to support yourself emotionally and financially?

Hip area

Grounding. Because of your pelvis connecting with your legs and feet. Creativity. Because your reproductive organs are housed in this area.

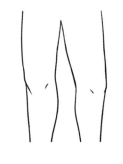

Legs

Walking on your path. What path are you walking on and how is the experience for you? Flexibility or rigidity in your attitudes can reflect in your knees. Can you allow yourself to be weak at the knees or overcome by feelings at times? Can you allow yourself to fall in love or be swept away by nature's beauty, for example? Thighs are powerful muscles, which help you to jump, run and bound. Thighs work together with core strength to help you feel strong. How strong have you been feeling lately?

Feet

Your feet walk in your shoes; they walk on your path. As part of your legs they are the closest to the ground, metaphorically representing the life path that you are walking on, how you feel about it and how grounded you have been. For example, have you stubbed your toe while in a hurry, or had to dig in your heels? Or perhaps you have felt a need to walk on eggshells around someone who you find challenging? Or perhaps you feel you would rather walk on a different path than the one you are on?

3) COME UP WITH A CONSTRUCTIVE RESPONSE

Consider how to make more space in your life for what might be needed, coming up with ideas and practical steps for how to go about it. How could your symptom point to a shift in attitude or a shift in focus in your life? Try asking yourself something about your growth from this experience, such as, 'If I could learn from this in some way, what could it teach me?' If you cannot think of anything then maybe you are being asked to trust life or to surrender trying to control everything, and to simply go with the flow. This process is all about tuning in to a constructive, optimistic frame of mind. You could also consider, 'If this makes perfect sense in my life at this point, what sense could that be?'

At some point you want to translate your new thoughts and personal learning opportunities into actions to help you realise change. You might consider if there are particular steps you can take in your life to help you integrate something of the life lesson, perhaps support you might seek, or investing in healthy habits such as exercise, meditation or the food you choose. In your body you might notice how you might be carrying tensions or discomfort. You could bring caring attention to these areas by, for example, loosening them up, breathing into them and stretching them out to free up restriction. You could also play with breathing an inspiring quality through you, like patience, kindness or courage, and notice how this changes your posture and mind.

You might consider what was happening for you when your symptom started and what you needed, then, what you might still need. Or, if something happens out of the blue, you might open to the possibility that life may be leading you in a new direction that could open new doors, even if you can't see how, yet.

'There is always gold to be mined in every experience' says Debbie Ford in her book *The Dark Side of the Light Chasers*. She shares that, with awareness and time, every wound holds wisdom and every misfortune can hold blessings. It may just take time to uncover what these blessings might be. The 'gold' that Ford speaks of, could be knowing yourself better, opening to trust or love or living more in line with your truth. It could be commitment to new honesty, perseverance, living life to the full, or anything else that feels true for you.

⇉ MINDFUL BODY MOMENT ⇇

Sensing the possibility for full body vitality in support of symptom management

Imagine climbing into a glistening bodysuit made of light, comfortable and sparkly material. Even draw the glistening bodysuit over your head, noticing that you can see through it and breathe easily in it. Now your whole body is snugly contained in this comfortable sparkle. From there, absorb the glittery feeling of it into your body, as if breathing it in so that your whole being glistens, right down to your cells. Spend extra time if you wish, absorbing the sparkle into the parts of your body that might be troubling you now, to encourage them to open to some sparkling support. Then spend a few moments experiencing your shiny body as a whole. To help you here, you could move awareness through your body to greet each glistening part in turn, from head down to toe. Perhaps look at different parts of your body in wonder as you imagine seeing and sensing your body's sparkling glow. In the words of Dr Candace Pert, 'Your mind is in every cell of your body.' Imagining your whole body glistening in this way can wake a sense of vitality at a cellular level, full of the potential for a glistening life.

Now bring your attention to a part of your body that might be hurting or ailing. Notice how it is surrounded by your glistening body and how it too is invited to glisten. Feeling the hurt contextualised in this full body way can remind you of the health that exists in the parts of you that are well. Perhaps you can feel into the possibility that your ailing parts are held and supported by the parts of your body that are well.

You might consider how this kind of whole-body perspective can perhaps change something about how your hurt, or ailing, part feels, or how you hold your body, or how you walk or move. Some people find that this type of visualisation can ease their pain and suffering because they can stop fixating on the hurt and instead open themselves to a bigger picture of their body and mind. What value might this add for you?

Even when we are ailing or injured, we can still pause to celebrate the vitality that we can experience. It is the vitality that can tingle, breathe and pulse brilliantly through us, no matter how some parts of us might feel. Doing so can offer some relief and new perspective. Perhaps it can also spark something in our life force to come to our aid.

Hold whatever your sense is of full-body glistening and vitality for a few more moments to really soak up the experience. Then, as you feel ready, return to your day.

⇒ MINDFUL BODY PROCESS ⇐

A visualisation for connecting with a 'higher' message

There are times when our experience is so challenging that soul-searching is called for. Perhaps you need to take time out to consider your priorities. What are the things you really want to do in your life that you might have put off? Now might be the time to make space for them. These can be times for big questions and possibly changes too. There are also times when we need to give up trying to find the answers or figure things out. These times we perhaps need to let go and see where our lives might lead us, all the while being open to guidance from wherever it may come.

To facilitate an experience of soul-searching, I have included a visualisation that you might find helpful. To carry it out, first sit comfortably in a quiet place where you can be uninterrupted for at least 10–15 minutes.

THE VISUALISATION

Picture yourself sitting quietly in a favourite, comfortable place. Notice your surroundings and how you feel being there. Imagine the sights, smells and sounds and the temperature of the air. Notice as much as you can. Let the scene come alive. When you feel ready, visualise becoming one with the energy of your surroundings. Visualise lightwaves branching further and further out into the universe. Awaken your heart and do your best to radiate love, compassion and gratitude outwards on these lightwaves, to fill the whole space around you. If this is difficult for you, you can simply imagine surrounding yourself with white, soothing light. Be with this experience for a few moments. If it is meaningful to you, invite a spiritual figure to join you there, perhaps feel your God in the space, or a spirit guide, guardian angel or helpful ancestor.

Ask out into this space, 'Is there a message for me?' Wait, listen and feel. Be open to what you might receive in word, feeling or image. Spend a few moments allowing this to unfold. Absorb your message in whatever form it comes. Then reflect for a few more moments, considering what this message could mean in your life now.

When you are ready, notice the outline of your physical body. Letting go of the visualisation, notice your body sitting in the space that you are currently in. Notice your posture and your breathing. Stretch and move your body to further ground you. If you wish, write down your experience or express it creatively or artistically in some way. Use this exercise whenever you wish. In it, your physicality, with all of its complaints, can feel like it dissolves into a vast, shared, universal sea of pure energy. It can offer respite when you are suffering – physically or emotionally. For some, consulting the energetic or spiritual dimension in this kind of way is soothing and meaningful. Others may appreciate a more concrete approach for engaging with their experience. Use whatever works for you.

CHAPTER 10

Mindful Body Moving: The Life Skill of Natural Movement

Your body has its own inherently positive direction and force...
Your body knows the direction of healing and life.

EUGENE GENDLIN

⇝ NATURAL MOVEMENT: A PATH TO PERSONAL GROWTH ⇜

One way of working through your body to cultivate greater vitality and instil consistent mindful body awareness is by practising moving naturally with your feelings and impulses, on a body level. When you are feeling stressed, sore or unwell, or when your emotions are hurting, following your natural movement, even for a few moments, can offer surprising relief and open you to fresh resourcefulness. In this way you can connect more deeply with yourself and consider what you need, from your body's perspective. You might discover deeper breathing or you might feel drawn to stretch out some parts of your body that hold tension, or apply some supportive touch, or shake or sway or reach your arms up, or curl up tight or stand like a statue. There is no right or wrong. This movement can shift how you feel and think. It can also build your sense of vitality. If you follow your natural movement, even for just a few minutes, you can feel more energised and in touch with yourself in a deeper way than usual.

As we learn to live more in touch with our authentic body movement and discover our ability to be with, and witness, our body in all of its changing expressions, it can translate into greater authenticity in all aspects of life. It can offer a constructive, empowering way to live with our emotional ups and downs. It can also be a path to personal growth when we notice our bodies with curiosity instead of criticism, and open to a whole sensory world inside us. Being open to our bodies can teach us about ourselves and guide as in times of need. One example of this benefit is expressed by Karen Whalen and Glenn Fleisch in their article that examines the connection between quantum physics principles and body awareness. They suggest that any time we observe something (in this case the body), it changes the nature of it.

> *Whenever we observe any part of the body or field of experiencing in an accepting, open, curious, and precise way, the quantum properties of its atoms and electrons, and their conglomerations into molecules, and on into molecular structures (like proteins, enzymes, parasites, viruses, cells, neurons, hormones, etc) are mobilised. As a result the cells will fire in new ways and will therefore affect the macrostructure and functioning of tissues, organs, bones, posture and psyche.*

In this article, Whalen explains that when she brought curious attention to her broken kneecap, while also holding awareness of her body as a whole, she was able to fully recover from her injury, even though she was over 50 years old at the time. In her words:

When I offer my knee an awareness of itself, connected to an awareness of the ankle, the shin, the feet, the thigh above it, (and) the hip joint, the firing activity of the knee discovers how it is or is not firing and can now synchronise itself with the firing of the whole leg. The knee itself, in its wisdom, knows how to connect with the whole leg and body. By simply noticing my knee, it naturally makes its own connections with the whole organism.

The same can apply to whatever we might be holding on to in our emotional bodies, such as an emotional challenge that we hold in a particular way. We can perhaps relate to it differently and shed new light on the matter when we locate it as part of a full body experience, identifying how the particular emotion lives, moves and evolves. Following our bodies can also feel like tuning into our souls as we connect with ourselves on a deeper level.

To access this enquiry into body and soul through natural movement, try not to organise movement; rather, just let it happen by following the movement that is already inside you. At first it might seem difficult to listen inwards to your body. Gradually you can come to notice how your body is constantly shifting, adjusting and expressing everything about your experience at the time. This includes responding to thoughts, feelings and general body sensations as well as to deep yearnings, needs or dreams that you might not even be aware of.

Our ability to influence our experience is what allows us to partner with, and support, our internal world. Trusting this process and investing time tuning in to this inner-body world is what can offer us a pathway to personal growth.

⇒ TWO OPTIONS FOR APPLYING NATURAL MOVEMENT IN YOUR LIFE ⇐

To follow are two ways that you can apply natural movement in your life. The first is called 'Anywhere, anytime exploring body feedback'. It is a way to pick up on daily body feedback that you can do inconspicuously if you need to, anywhere and anytime – even sitting in an office with other people around you. You might be surprised how quickly this kind of exploration can energise you. You may also feel relieved at having acknowledged your feelings in this visceral, sensory way.

The second way that you can apply natural movement in your life is by dedicating time to it, referred to here as 'setting up a moving ritual'. This application is for when you have some time and privacy to follow your natural movement more fully. You might do this for a few minutes at home – perhaps as a way to unwind at the end of your day. Or you could include it as much as feels appropriate, before or after an exercise session. Or you could practise your moving ritual for a few minutes at the start of your day to connect with your authenticity. When you are going through a challenging time emotionally, you can perhaps make some extra time for this practice, which can potentially bring you relief, support and a helpful perspective.

ANYWHERE ANYTIME EXPLORING BODY FEEDBACK

Here is the first of the two ways for incorporating mindful, natural movement into your day. This one helps you to pick up on body feedback, when you notice it, for the sake of freeing up energy, releasing tension, acknowledging feelings and perhaps clearing your mind to focus on what you need to. You can explore the messages carried in your body's posture and movement at any time, in any place, and whether you are sitting or standing. Let's say you are sitting and find that your leg is jiggling and you are, to some extent, holding your breath; you would pick one action at a time for exploration. Once you have chosen which action to start with you hold your focus on it for a few moments, becoming curious about its energy and what it might be communicating about your state of mind. To help you focus on it, you could exaggerate or intensify the movement so that you can feel it more noticeably. What is its energy? What is its quality of movement? Experiment with following this action for a few moments, allowing your body to have a mind of its own. You might notice that your jiggling leg has a 'desire' to run away or escape that could apply to some situation you are in. To explore this you could exaggerate the movement in your legs as much as feels appropriate, perhaps moving your legs and feet around a bit to explore how your body is expressing this energy. Perhaps you can shake your legs out or go for a short walk to get your legs moving. Perhaps doing so increases your energy level, or perhaps it shifts your attitude in some way. Consider how you feel as you acknowledge your body's expression of these feelings. Sometimes all your body needs is to be listened to and acknowledged, which could feel relieving.

If you still notice your breathing is shallow, you can go on to acknowledge this, too. You might notice that there is tightness in your chest that 'wishes' to contract along with your abdomen. Allow your body to follow through with this movement impulse as much as you feel comfortable. You might notice that the energy of this spreads into a desire to tighten your hands into fists and perhaps clench your jaw tightly, too. These actions might give you different information about your attitudes than your leg jiggling. Perhaps this is a message about a need to be in control, or about frustration or anger that you might not have been focusing on but that is bottled up and simmering beneath the surface. What does this part of you need and how might you respond to this need now? You might feel like taking a deep breath or massaging areas that feel tense (the first chapter on greeting your body with touch can give you some ideas), to relieve tension. Or you might feel a need to act in some way, like picking up the phone to speak with someone or calling a meeting to address something bothering you. Respecting that your body language holds valuable feedback about your attitudes or your situation, gives you the power to notice and respond sooner to what you need, instead of allowing stresses and strains to accumulate.

SETTING UP A MOVING RITUAL

This is the Mindful Body Moving practice for when you have more time and privacy to follow your natural movement fully. To practise natural movement in this way, dedicate some time to it – perhaps 5 or 10 minutes to start – and as you become familiar with it you might choose to practise for longer. Find a time of day that works for you. Some people like to do a few minutes before a regular exercise routine or towards the end of the day to help unwind and acknowledge feelings from the day. Or you could use it with a few gentle stretches first thing in the morning, to set an authentic tone for your day. Or when you have a moment to yourself and you are feeling stressed or bothered, you can experiment with following your body for a few moments to notice what this might offer you.

During this time you are invited to follow how your body wants to move. Some find it helpful, before freely following their natural movement, to start with a head-to-toe body greeting. This can allow you to use awareness, movement, touch or breathing to each part of your body, to awaken greater body presence. This can also help you to notice which part of your body, or what feelings inside you, draw your attention. This will become the starting point for the natural movement exploration to follow.

To mark the start and end of your unstructured natural movement exploration, take one or two deep breaths. This is helpful for your body to feel contained in the process and can also give a sense of completion at the end as you mark the end of your exploration with one or two deep breaths.

Try closing your eyes as you explore your movement. Closing your eyes will help reduce self-consciousness and connect you internally. You could also move naturally, with your eyes open, if you prefer.

Listen to your body and notice how it wants to move. Follow your feelings, sensations and impulses towards this movement. Explore your curiosity about a part of your body or a body symptom, such as a twinge, or the sense of your energy level, or an ache or restlessness or tension in some part of you. Then you are invited to follow your feelings or impulses. Move into your body with curiosity about how it shapes you and how it is alive and constantly in motion. You can follow your natural breathing that is closely connected with your emotions, allowing your breathing to move and shape your body organically. You could also start with an image, for example if you remember something from a dream, and feel into how your body shapes around a particular image and then you can begin exploring the imagery through your movement from there. Or you can start moving without a particular focus. If you feel tired and heavy, slump down; if you feel energised, let it spring outwards from you in a way that feels authentic. If a part of your body draws your attention at any point during your exploration, follow it.

You can follow any movement impulse to see where it leads you and then move on to explore the next thing that you become curious about. Don't try to move with yesterday's feelings – your natural movement will feel false. Follow what feels true in the moment. Be still if that is your truth, or lie down, sit, curl up or stand up, shake or move about. Then be open to how your desire for movement develops from there.

Follow whatever feelings and energy are really there, as if this were meditation in motion. There really is no prescribed route when following your natural movement and it can be done for a few moments or for as long as you wish at any time during your day.

If you are not sure what to do, you might watch or think of young children at play and you will see full body expression in motion. You were like that once and you carry the memory inside you of being carefree and expressive like a child. Doing so can feel novel and unusual, to start with, and very natural as you continue. Ultimately the aim is to incorporate natural movement more and more into your life, as an expression of your authenticity. This obviously does not mean that you need to act like a child when you are out and about; it simply means you make some time, even as little as five minutes a day (perhaps longer when you are working through a personal challenge) to tune in to, and follow, your body for all that it can offer you. These offerings include energy, authenticity and feeling connected with your truth. The more regularly you practise, the more this authenticity will spill over into your daily life.

Find a satisfying way to end for the time being, knowing that you can return to your explorations another time. If you are holding something challenging and it is time to close your exploration, you can ask your mind or body to come up with a helpful, supportive image, or movement direction. Give yourself a few moments to embody and develop this exploration before moving on with your day. Some ideas are: to surround yourself in a bubble of safety or to consider a helpful word, like courage or trust, and spend a few moments moving with the quality of the word as you encourage yourself to embody something of that quality to help you when you might be feeling vulnerable. If you do not feel complete, at least you honored your experience, which might be energising no matter how far along you get with your process. You can always continue your exploration another time.

To get a sense of feeling complete on a body level, think of yawning, as you would on waking up in the morning, with a good stretch, similar to how a cat or dog would. Try it out. Invite yourself to yawn and give your body a good stretch to go with it. You know when the stretch feels complete. It is when you feel complete and ready to move on from it. It feels satisfying to follow through with movement to its natural conclusion. The action releases muscular or nervous system energy in the process. This sense of sequencing movement through to completion can also happen during your natural movement exploration. With this in mind you can explore bringing your movement to a close in a way that feels satisfying. Sometimes you may not feel complete, that is OK, too. Life is a continuous flow of energy and movement that might find resolution in other ways as you move through the rest of your day. There are also times when our processes are in progress for days and weeks, or months at a time, in which case our movement might reflect this ongoing nature and we can come to accept not feeling fully complete. Perhaps we can then seek out feeling 'complete enough' for the time being. There is no right and wrong, just what feels true. So we can learn to move with whatever comes up for us in the endless cycles of movement in life.

To end, take a deep breath to mark your conclusion. If your eyes were closed, open them slowly and consciously as if seeing your surroundings anew. If you feel like it, journalise or draw something from your process. Then be open to how you might carry your authentic movement forwards with you into your day and what value it might bring to you.

There might be times when you wish you could explore natural movement spontaneously, like when you are out and you get emotionally triggered. To respect social appropriateness you can also follow through with your body's natural movement, in your imagination, perhaps with some minimal physical movement. This way you can engage with your body and its messages at any time that you wish. For example, as an outlet for emotional energy you might visualise how your body wishes to respond in movement to acknowledge and perhaps evolve your experience in a helpful direction.

You might also embody some of this movement in another inconspicuous way, such as representing a feeling in just your hand and letting your hand shape around, and process, your feelings through its movement. This can give you an on-the-spot way to stay connected with your body and its natural movement. For example, if you have a headache, you might express its energy in your fists. Spend a few moments focusing on the energy in your hand, listening for feedback about your headache. This action can possibly offer you some on-the-spot relief. Or if you feel anxious, perhaps before a presentation, for example, you could take a few moments to shake your body out as inconspicuously or conspicuously as you feel comfortable or to place a hand on your chest for some acknowledgement of your feelings and support. The invitation, even when carried out inconspicuously, is to follow what your body feels like it needs to help you feel calmer and more contained.

In these kinds of ways you take the time to connect and engage with the ebb and flow of life as expressed through your body. With practice, some aspire to this being a constant way of life, while others choose to dip in now and again. The choice is yours.

⇒ WHEN HELP IS NEEDED ⇐

For some of us, tuning into and following the life of our bodies can be a smooth process. For others who have endured much suffering there can be resistance to looking inwards. It simply can feel too unsafe to tap into what is there. In these cases professional support is recommended before using natural movement on your own. Examples of when you might need assistance could be when you try out the practice and it causes more distress than support. This can be the case when you have a history of trauma, chronic depression, anxiety, or other psychiatric or medical conditions that cause pain and distress. In these cases, you might require support in building some internal strength and resources to be able to feel safe in, and appreciative of, your internal world.

⇒ THE VALUE OF BODY AWARENESS ⇐

Whenever you spend time being aware of your body in a sensing, non-thinking kind of way (as opposed to judging it), more and more neural connections are activated in a part of the brain called the insula. The insula facilitates your felt experience of mind-body integration and can be stimulated any time you move your body's joints (the moveable parts of your body). Take a moment to experiment with this by bringing some movement to the joints of your body, exploring bending, rotating and moving your arms, legs and spine. You might notice that moving even a little brings you more in touch with your body because you are increasing the blood flow to, and oxygenation of, more parts of your body, including your brain. This means more energy and more physical comfort, perhaps, because you are more conscious of how you are sitting or standing. It can also refresh your ability to focus.

Activity in the insula is stimulated any time we move our bodies. This happens when we exercise (such as running, swimming, going to the gym or doing Yoga), or when we dance or play actively. It is also stimulated when we quietly attend to our breathing and body sensations, such as when meditating as well as any time we use a Mindful Body Moment from this book.

Part of each insula's job (there are two insulae, one on each side of the brain) is to allow you to track the internal state of your body. You can see this as two eyes in your brain, looking inwards. When you attend to the internal state of your body regularly, research has shown that the insulae actually thicken from the increase in neural activity and neural connections made inside it. This makes it easier for you to feel connected with your body. The insulae are also involved in the sensing of emotions. So when the insulae are well developed they help to increase self-awareness and the ability to be in touch with your feelings. Related to this is a connection between the insula and empathy. As we can sense our own internal world, so we become better at sensing the internal world of others, which is the foundation for empathy. In the brain it is found that the same neural circuits light up when we are sensing our own feelings and the feelings of others. When we attune to how others are feeling, the brain seems to recognise feelings as one and the same, no matter if they originate in our experience or another's. So by building up your insula and becoming more skilled with mind-body integration, you can become both self-aware and more empathic because the two go hand-in-hand.

Even when our history has been painful, the skill of being able to look inwards can offer us a slow path back to feeling alive and in control again. Trauma expert Dr Bessel van der Kolk speaks of psychological health in terms of feeling fluid and alive. In his book *The Body Keeps The Score,* he relays the value of developing interoception as part of a recovery process from trauma. Interoception is the ability to feel impulses towards movement. In doing so we can become aware of how our inner world constantly interacts with our thoughts and emotions. Dr van der Kolk advocates physical practices like Yoga and martial arts to support trauma recovery because of how they improve body awareness.

⇉ OTHER WAYS TO CONNECT WITH NATURAL RHYTHMS ⇇

Besides moving to the music of your body's internal world, you can also put on actual music and move, hum or sing. This is another way to awaken your vibrant body energy. Bopping to a beat or swaying to a gentle melody is age-old medicine for your soul.

Spending time in nature is another naturally uplifting, refreshing reminder of your human nature. Sit by a forest stream with the soothing sounds of water and birds chirping, or on a rock by the powerful ocean; spend time in whatever natural scene speaks most to you. Allow nature to plug you back into your essential self and your sensory aliveness.

Cultivating vitality and following natural impulses also requires listening to other ways that your body gives you feedback. Simple things like resting when you feel tired, getting up and out when you are awake, eating until you are satisfied, choosing healthy foods and other sensible ways to take care of your body and mind, are all effective. But even these seemingly simple things can be immensely challenging with the rigorous demands of modern living, work commitments and family. Fortunately there is an in-built incentive in doing the best that we can with this, which is the reward of how good we can feel when we do honor our body's natural rhythms and needs. Gifts include health, energy, clarity of mind, greater enjoyment of life and the experience of our body as a rich and rewarding place to live from.

CHAPTER 11

Natural Vital Conclusions

There is a natural order and harmony to this world, which we can discover. But we cannot just study that order scientifically or measure it mathematically. We have to feel it – in our bones, in our hearts, in our minds.

CHÖGYAM TRUNGPA RINPOCHE

This conclusion brings us home to nature. Throughout the book you have been invited to sink your awareness down into your mindful body, using different approaches and focusing on applying them in different ways. Life slows down to a more natural pace that paradoxically is dynamic and full of energy in its grounded, vital way. In this you can connect with yourself as an integral part of nature with a natural intelligence and vital energy, down to the microscopic level of every cell of your body. As you tune in to your natural rhythms you can also wake up to a sense of purpose and place. This can feel balancing, inspiring and deeply energising. It can also be an antidote to the stressful effects of fast-paced living.

It is important to honour our thinking, also needed for a balanced, healthy life. Thinking adds analysis, reason, creativity, planning and assigning meaning, to day-to-day experience. But it is by sensing our lives in a vital, open-hearted way that we can remember our true nature. This is a source of nourishment for our mental and physical health. Thinking only becomes a problem when we forget that we are an integral part of nature. Luckily we cannot stay separated from nature for long. Our bodies have a way of calling our attention via their constant feedback, in the form of emotional or physical aches and pains in response to stressful ways of living. If you neglect your body then it is experienced as your opponent. If you follow your body, it becomes your ally.

⇒ VITAL ENERGY ⇐

Life is forever unfolding, pulsing, becoming and receding from the core of our cells through to our full body experience of it. By noticing and following the dynamic energy that lives beneath the surface of regular awareness, we can also become dynamic and energised with life. This experience is both electric and fluid and it is constantly changing from moment to moment. When we are full of this kind of vital energy it is also as if we are tuning in to something bigger, perhaps the entire electromagnetic field of the earth as a giant matrix that connects everyone and everything. Vital energy is said to originate in this vast field of energy that we all draw from and that animates our uniqueness. It is vital energy available to everyone and belonging to no one and, in the words of Albert Einstein, it 'cannot be created or destroyed, it can only be changed from one form to another.'

An ultimate gift of body awareness is a natural connection to abundant vital energy. According to Arnold Mindell, the energy that can be generated through proprioceptive and kinesthetic awareness, or awareness of body sensations, movement and even your impulses towards movement, builds 'body power'. 'Body power' is another term for vital energy. People who cultivate their relationship with this vital energy can radiate immense vitality and energy. Mindell also offers that following your body is like following lost parts of your soul. He speaks of how, in time, your body can begin to feel like a dreaming body that is deeply connected with yourself and your soul. When feeling connected in this way you can find yourself filled with energy. Then all that is left is to listen inwards and direct that energy outwards to contribute to your own life as well as to our communities and our world.

⇒ NATURAL INTELLIGENCE, A PATH TO SELF-REALISATION ⇐

All around us we can see nature fulfilling itself, from the tiny acorn becoming a giant oak tree, to a small weed finding its way to the light through six inches of concrete. Life is constantly aiming at its own fruition. We are the only ones who (can) hold ourselves back from fulfillment, for the very essence of our being is already free.
Debbie Shapiro, *The Bodymind Workbook*

To follow are a few points for your reflection. What stage of your natural growth are you in now? Have you planted some new seeds in some areas of your life? Are you harvesting the bounty in other areas? What does your fruition look like? If you are an acorn now or if a while ago you started out as one, what is the 'oak tree' that you are maturing towards? Feel and imagine what your 'oak tree' might be like as the mature expression of yourself, perhaps representing your legacy as the unique expression of your vital energy in the world. Is there a message in this for your current self? Consider this for a few moments.

Even the natural progression from birth through to inevitable death can be embraced with grace and flow. We can remain timelessly open-hearted with each stage of our lives. Each stage has its own offerings of beauty, strength and vulnerability for us to hold and express. Each stage is its own rich, natural journey and adventure, and its own authentic expression. So we can experience self-realisation at each stage of our lives even when dying. We can approach even this very last stage with the same awareness and flow, awe and heartfelt presence as we approach the rest of our living.

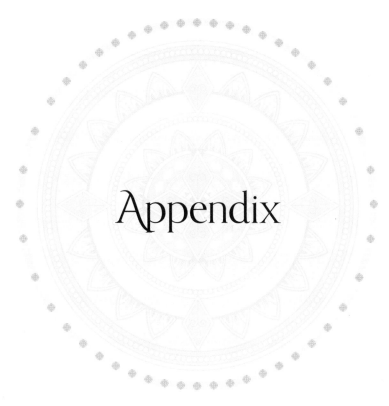

Appendix

⇒ MINDFULNESS WITH A BODY FOCUS: TWO DAILY PRACTICE OPTIONS ⇐

To follow are two mindfulness practices that draw on your body as a resource for living in the present moment. They can guide you to being more grounded, wise and centred in life, naturally opening your awareness to the present moment, to your inherent vitality and to being more open-minded. The more you practise, the more this state of body mindfulness can become your new normal.

Both practices are designed to be easy to incorporate into a busy life. The first practice guides you to run awareness through your body from head to toe, which can have a relaxing effect. The second practice guides you to run awareness upwards through your body from feet to head, which can have an energising effect. Both options end with an invitation to tune in to your heart for a warm, loving tone to carry forwards.

HOW TO USE THE PRACTICES

These practices can be carried out in just a minute or two once you have learned them, and can be applied anywhere and anytime, even while you are waiting in the shopping line or stuck in traffic! You can also take longer with them as dedicated body-based mindfulness practices if you wish to deepen your experience. To do so, either move awareness more slowly through your body, or you could repeat the option that you prefer a few times, to reinforce the effect.

CONNECTING WITH YOUR BODY IN A CALM, RELAXING WAY

This practice can be carried out with eyes closed for a deeper, meditative effect or with eyes open, especially when applied on the spot and in the course of your day. As a dedicated mindfulness practice it is recommended that you find a quiet space to sit, at a time of day that works best for you, such as in the morning, to set a mindful tone for the day, or in the evening to help you de-stress. Used in this way it is recommended that you close your eyes to help you focus in on your body.

What to do

Sit (or stand) comfortably. Keep your eyes open while you read these instructions and if you are out and about using the practice. Once you are familiar with the practice, closing your eyes such as when using the practice meditatively, can enhance its effectiveness.

Notice your breath. Breathe naturally.

Feel air passing into and out of your nostrils.

Keep your focus on your upper lip and the insides of your nostrils.

Feel air passing in and out over this area.

Remain focused on the feeling for a few moments of your breathing as it moves into and out of your nostrils.

If your mind begins to wander, with kindness when you notice, let it return to your breathing.

Then imagine your body as a sponge.

Run awareness like warm water slowly and steadily through your sponge body from the top of your head down to the tips of your fingers and toes. (If you do not like a water image, you can choose to run awareness like soothing light through your body or simply to move your awareness through your body from head to toe, noticing sensations in each part as you go along.) Spend a few moments with each body area as your awareness soaks into it. Feel into the sensations and vitality that you might be able to contact in each part.

Starting with awareness to the top of your head, soak awareness into this area. Then move your awareness downwards to your face and the back of your head, spending a few moments allowing your awareness to penetrate. Experience the feeling of life and fullness in this area. Then move your awareness to your lower face, jaw and the base of your head and on down through your neck. Then into your shoulders and down into your upper arms, elbows, lower arms, wrists, hands and fingers. Then soak awareness into your chest area, front and back and on down through to your diaphragm and on into your lower torso, soaking awareness into your abdominal and lower back area. Continue downwards into your hip area and pelvic bowl and on down into your upper legs, knees, lower legs, ankles, feet and toes, soaking each part of your body with your awareness and with curiosity. To end, let your awareness expand to include your body as a whole, drenched or filled with your awareness and a sense of full body vitality. Spend a few moments with this experience of your body as a warm, full and grounded whole.

Sitting with this fuller sense of your body, gently smile. Feel love warming and spreading through you, inviting your whole body to smile along with you. Then spread heartfelt warmth outwards to the space around you, warming and radiating outwards. Take a few moments to imagine sharing this loving glow with anyone who needs it. Then expand loving feelings further outwards into the world in an expansive warm glow. When you feel ready, take a deep breath and stretch your body before moving out into your day or night.

Note that, for a longer mindfulness practice, and to increase the meditative effect, you can expand on this exercise. You can simply move awareness more slowly through your body from head to toe. You could also follow the head-to-toe awareness with gradually moving your awareness back up your body from toes through to head. Then you would alternate moving awareness from head to toe and toe to head as many times as you wish for a longer, deeper practice. Use the smile and focusing on your heart's warm glow just once at the end, to mark the close of your meditation.

CONNECTING WITH YOUR BODY IN AN ENERGISING WAY

This practice works best standing, although it can be carried out sitting, too, if you wish. In this practice you keep your eyes open and move awareness upwards through your body from toes up to head. As you go along you are invited to greet and feel into each part of your body. You can use any method that works for you to wake up each body part. You might use breath, movement, tensing and relaxing, touch or brief massage, or perhaps stretching or shaking out the different areas. In the process, you enhance your body awareness while perhaps generating warmth and a tingle of vitality in different parts and in your body as a whole.

You can use this practice absolutely any time. You might add it to your warm-up before exercising, or as a way to wake up your body at the start of each day, perhaps spending longer with certain parts of your body that might need more support on the day. As with the previous practice, you can also use this practice anywhere and anytime, even while waiting in the shopping line or sitting in traffic, to help you feel more energised and to help clear your mind.

What to do

Breathe naturally as you go through the process.

To start, drop your awareness into your toes and feet, moving, wriggling, stretching out, tensing and relaxing or using any method you like to wake up your awareness of this part of your body. Move awareness gradually up to greet, move and feel into your ankles and then your lower legs, your knees, upper legs and hips. Greet your lower torso including your abdomen and lower back, followed by your upper torso including the front and back sides of your chest front, and on up to your shoulders, neck, face and head. Notice, and perhaps touch or move the different parts of your face and all the way up to your scalp and hair. Then bring awareness and movement to your fingers, feeling how they are filled with life, too, then gradually move on to greet, move and feel into your hands, wrists and forearms, elbows and upper arms and on up to your shoulders, noticing the sense of life in each part in turn.

Now feel the connection between your arms and your shoulders by using some movement to feel how they are connected and how they can move together. Move on to feeling the connection between your shoulders and hips, noticing how movement in your shoulders connects with movement in your hips and how movement in your hips and shoulders together can release tension in your torso, such as releasing your solar plexus area (the bundle of nerves that can create a knot of tension in your core). Spend a few moments now with your spine, from your tailbone up to the top of your neck. Breathe into, move or stretch out your spine to enhance your awareness and sense of vitality in this area.

Following this, turn your mindful attention to your body as a whole. Feel the connections between all parts of your body and how your whole body can feel integrated as a whole. You can use movement or stillness, breath or stretching or whatever feels good, to bring your whole body alive in your awareness. Is there a part of your body that needs a little more care and attention? If so, give this part of you a few more moments of attention and then return to your sense of your body as a whole.

Plant your feet evenly on the ground before closing this body mindfulness practice. Spend a few moments quietly feeling the rhythm of life breathing and pulsing in and through every cell of your body. Experience or sense the life of your body as a whole.

Then smile, even just a small smile, inviting your whole body to smile along with you. Spread warm feelings outwards and, if you wish, hold in mind those you love, or someone who might benefit from your love today.

When you feel ready, take a deep breath and a final stretch, or perhaps place your hand over your heart or over a part of your body that needs support, as a way to mark the close of your body greeting, for now.

Acknowledgments

Thank you to my husband, Stephen, for all your enormous and loving support. Without you my self-confidence would be half of what it is. Thank you also to our daughters Emmah and Miela for pure love and for all the learning, growing and playing together.

I gratefully acknowledge all my teachers at Naropa University where I studied my Masters degree in Somatic Psychology. I want to mention two teachers who were key to the work that I have taken forward. The first is Dr Christine Caldwell who was my core teacher at Naropa and whose book *Getting Our Bodies Back* is one of the much-loved textbooks for the courses that I run. The second is Zoe Avstreih, for a wonderful method for working with dreams as well as for introducing me to the practice of Authentic Movement. I am also grateful for the Naropa system, as a whole, that steeped me in many mindful, embodied and heartfelt approaches for understanding psychology and promoting wellbeing.

The opportunity to work with hundreds of open-minded and stimulating students, as well as my work with private psychotherapy clients, was a big inspiration for writing this book. Thank you to you all. Thank you also to the founder of the South African College of Applied Psychology (SACAP), Marc Feitelberg for the opportunity in 2005 to design and go on to teach the somatic counseling skills training module for over a decade, as part of their counseling, coaching and psychology curricula.

I would like to thank my mother who many years ago helped me to realise my first dream of becoming a professional dancer and then my second dream too, of studying at Naropa University. I would also like to thank my father, sister and brother for all of your support and kindness.

Finally I would like to say thank you to the team at Rockpool Publishing for giving this book life out in the world and for welcoming me into the Rockpool family.

Sources and Notes

⇞ INTRODUCTION ⇝

Aposhyan, S. (1999). *Natural Intelligence: Body-Mind integration and human development.* Lippincott Williams & Wilkins: Baltimore, MD and (2007) Now Press: Boulder, Colorado

Doidge, N. (2007). *The Brain that Changes Itself: Stories of Personal Triumph from the Frontiers of Brain Science,* Chapter 9 (Turning Our Ghosts into our Ancestors). Penguin Group: South Africa, London

⇞ CHAPTER 1: GREETING YOUR BODY ⇝

Aposhyan, S. (1999). *Natural Intelligence: Body-Mind integration and human development.* Lippincott Williams & Wilkins: Baltimore, MD and (2007) Now Press: Boulder, Colorado

To refer to the work of Roz Carroll go to: www.thinkbody.co.uk/

Guerrero, L., Andersen, P.A. and Afifi, W. (2014). *Close Encounters: Communication in Relationships.* Sage Publications, Inc.: California

Mines, S. (2003). *We are all in shock: How overwhelming experiences shatter you.... And what you can do about it.* Career Press: USA

For research by the Touch Research Institute at the University of Miami School of Medicine, refer to www.miami.edu/touch-research/

⇒ CHAPTER 2: BRAINWAVES AND THE PLACE FOR BODY AWARENESS ⇐

To refer to the work of Richard Davidson go to: http://richardjdavidson.com

Killingsworth, M. A. and Gilbert, D. T. (2010). A Wandering Mind is an Unhappy Mind, *Science* (magazine), Volume 330, Issue 6006

Example of research by Dr Melinda Maxfield, PhD: Maxfield, Melinda. 'Effects of Rhythmic Drumming on EEG and Subjective Experience.' http://sica.stanford.edu/events/brainwaves/MaxfieldABSTRACT.pdf

⇒ CHAPTER 3: CHANGE YOUR POSTURE, CHANGE YOUR MIND ⇐

To see Amy Cuddy's TED talk: https://www.ted.com/talks/amy_cuddy_your_body_language_shapes_who_you_are

Examples of Richard Depue's work: His findings on dopamine's relationship to personality in the *Journal of Personality and Social Psychology* (1994, Vol. 67), on neurobiological factors in personality and depression in the *European Journal of Personality*(1995, Vol. 9). On the neurobiological implications for personality, emotion and personality disorder is found in the book edited by

Lenzenweger, M. and Clarkin, J. (1996). Title: *Major Theories of Personality Disorder.* The Guilford Press: New York and London

Fisher, H. (2010). *Why Him Why Her: How to find and keep lasting love.* Holt Paperbacks: New York

For examples of Dr Erik Peper's research refer to https://biofeedbackhealth.org/ archives/

To refer to the work of Dr Richard Petty, see: richardpettymd.com

⇛ CHAPTER 4: STRESS AND BODY FIRST-AID ⇚

Aposhyan, S. (1999). *Natural Intelligence: Body-Mind integration and human development.* Lippincott Williams & Wilkins: Baltimore, MD and (2007) by Now Press: Boulder, Colorado

Goleman, D. (1995). *Emotional Intelligence: Why it can matter more than IQ.* Bloomsbury Publishing: London

Goulston, M. (2009). *Just Listen Just Listen: Discover the Secret to Getting Through to Absolutely Anyone.* Amacom: USA

To view the work of Dr Matthew Lieberman, see http://lieberman.socialpsychology. org

Examples of Daniel J. Siegel's many books:

Siegel, D. J. (2011). *Mindsight: The New Science Of Personal Transformation.* Bantam Books Trade Paperbacks: New York

Siegel, D. J. (2012). *Pocket guide to interpersonal neurobiology: An integrative handbook of the mind.* W. W. Norton & Company: New York

⇛ CHAPTER 5: EMOTIONS AND TURNING TO THE BODY ⇚

Ford, D. (2001). *The Dark Side of the Light Chasers: Reclaiming Your Power, Creativity, Brilliance and Dreams.* Hodder & Stoughton: London

Pert, C. (2006). *Everything you need to know to feel go(o)d.* Hay House: California, London, Sydney, Johannesburg

Pert, C. (1999). *Molecules of Emotion: The Science behind Mind-Body Medicine.* Touchstone: New York

Weiser Cornell, A. (1996).*The Power of Focusing: A practical guide to emotional self-healing.* New Harbinger Publications: California

⇒ CHAPTER 6: MINDFUL BODY DREAMING ⇐

Example of Thomas Budzynski's work:

Budzynski, T.H., Budzynski, H.K., Evans, J.R. and Abarbanel, A. (2008). *Introduction to Quantitative EEG and Neurofeedback: Advanced Theory and Applications,* 2nd Edition. Elsevier: Netherlands

Epstein, G. (2004). *Waking Dream Therapy: Unlocking The Secrets of Self Through Dreams and Imagination.* ACMI Press

Siegel, D. J. (2010). *Mindsight: The New Science of Personal Transformation.* Random House: New York, USA

Taylor, J. (1993).*Where People Fly and Water Runs Uphill: Using Dreams to Tap the Wisdom of the Unconscious.* Grand Central Publishing: New York

To refer to the work of Montague Ullman, see: http://siivola.org/monte/

⇒ CHAPTER 7: OUR BODIES REMEMBER ⇐

Ainsworth, M. D. S., & Bowlby, J. (1991), An ethological approach to personality development. *American Psychologist, 46,* 331-341.

Note: Attachment Theory originates in the work of John Bowlby and Mary Ainsworth. Two examples of articles expanding on this theory are: http://www.psychology.sunysb.edu/attachment/online/inge_origins.pdf

Hazan, C., & Shaver, P. R. (1987). Romantic love conceptualised as an attachment process. *Journal of Personality and Social Psychology, 52,* 511-524.

Two examples of Dr Stephen Porge's work:

Porges, S. (2011). *The polyvagal theory: Neurophysiologial foundations of emotions, attachment, communication, and self-regulation.* New York: W. W. Norton & Company.

Porges, S.W. (1995). Orienting in a defensive world: Mammalian modifications of our evolutionary heritage. A Polyvagal Theory. Psychophysiology, 32, 301-318.

An example of Dr Lloyd Silverman's work:

Silverman, L.H. and Weinberger, J. Mummy and I are one: Implications for psychotherapy, *American Psychologist*, Vol 40(12), Dec 1985, 1296-1308. http://dx.doi.org/10.1037/0003-066X.40.12.1296

Dr. Thomas Verny has written many books and professional publications. He is the founder of the Association for Prenatal and Perinatal Psychology and Health (APPPAH) and Journal of Prenatal and Perinatal Psychology and Health. To find out more about Dr Verny's work, see: www.trvernymd.com

⇒ CHAPTER 8: HEALING OLD PATTERNS, ENHANCING VITALITY ⇐

To refer to the work of Dr Diane Poole Heller, see: https://dianepooleheller.com

To refer to the work of Dr Harville Hendrix, see: http://harvilleandhelen.com

Tatkin, S. (2012). *Wired for Love: How understanding your partner's brain can help you defuse conflict and spark intimacy.* New Harbinger Publications: California

To see Stan Tatkin's 'Welcome Home Hug': https://www.youtube.com/watch?v=V9FBdC2Kykg

⇒ CHAPTER 9: AILMENTS AND INJURIES AS METAPHORS FOR LIFE ⇐

Connelly, D. (1979). *Traditional Acupuncture: The Law of the Five Elements.* Centre for Traditional Acupuncture: University of California

⇒ CHAPTER 10: MINDFUL BODY MOVING: THE LIFE SKILL OF NATURAL MOVEMENT ⇐

For more information about methods referred to in the section on exploring body feedback, see: Caldwell, C. (1996). *Getting Our Bodies Back: Recovery and Transformation Through Body-Centered Psychotherapy.* Shambhala: Boston and London

Siegel, D. (2010). *The Mindful Therapist: A Clinician's Guide to Mindsight and Neural Integration.* W.W. Norton & Company: New York and London

van der Kolk, B. (2014). *The Body Keeps The Score: Brain, Mind, and Body in the Healing of Trauma.* Viking Books: USA

Whalen, K. and Fleisch, G. (2012). Quantum Consciousness: An explanatory model for life forward movement in whole body focusing (Part 1). *The Folio: A journal for Focusing and Experiential Therapy, Volume 23 (1), p.84-97* (specific quotes used in this chapter are on page 89)

Note that the section on Natural Movement adapts skills from the practice of Authentic Movement, applied in this case to exploring on one's own.

⇻ CHAPTER 11: NATURAL VITAL CONCLUSIONS ⇺

Mindell, A. (1993). *The Shaman's Body: A New Shamanism for Transforming Health, Relationships, and the Community.* Harper Collins Publishers: New York

Shapiro, D. (2002). *The Body Mind Workbook: Explaining How the Mind and Body Work Together.* Vega Publishing: London

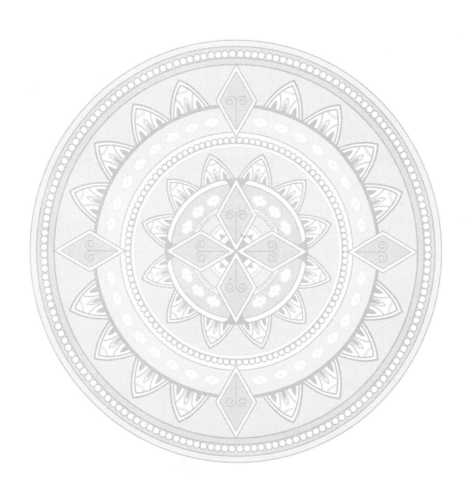

About the Author

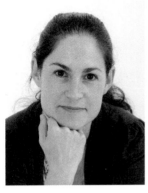

Noa holds a Masters degree in somatic (or body-mind) psychology through Naropa University, which is the birthplace of the modern mindfulness movement. Her background includes over a decade of teaching applied somatic psychology skills, running a private psychotherapy practice, being a published author on yoga and a former professional ballet dancer. She is the best-selling author of *The Yoga Handbook, Yoga: A union of mind and body* (Struik); and *Yoga for Ideal Weight and Shape* (New Holland Publishing and Juta Publishers). Her books have sold hundreds of thousands of copies worldwide and are translated into many languages.

Noa runs her own psychology practice that includes working with individuals, couples and groups. She also offers tailored talks and workshops in the corporate sector on topics such as stress management, emotional resilience and relationship management.

For more information, visit www.noabelling.com